pilates for weight loss

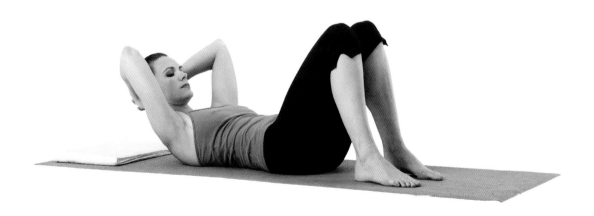

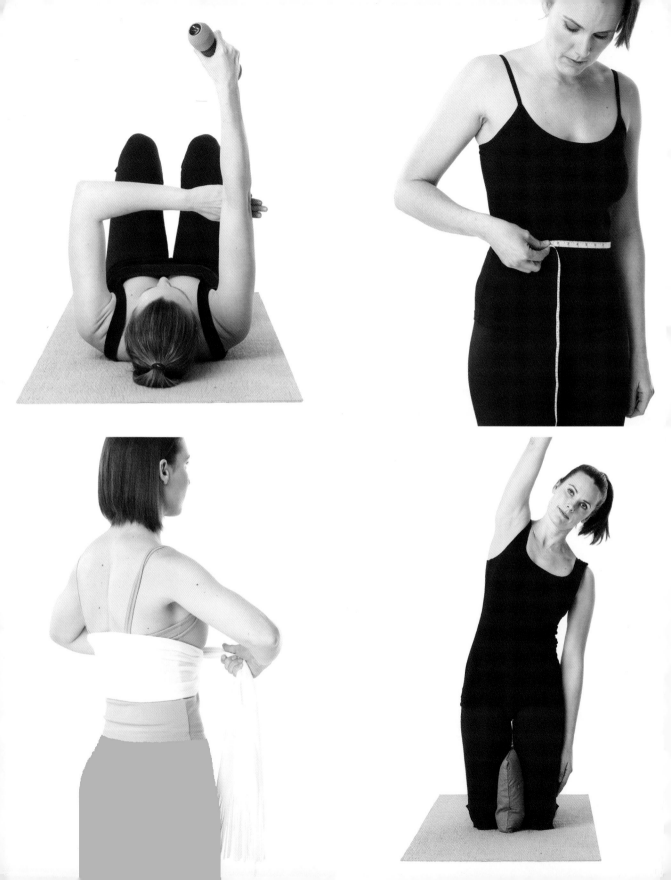

pilates
for weight loss

The fast, effective way to change
your body shape for good

Lynne Robinson

Photography by Eddie MacDonald

Kyle Cathie Limited

First published in Great Britain in 2008 by
Kyle Cathie Limited
23 Howland Street
London W1T 4AY
www.kylecathie.com

This edition first published in 2011

ISBN 978 0 85783 013 5

A Cataloguing in Publication record for this title is available
from the British Library.

Printed and bound in China by C&C Offset Printing Company Ltd

Project editor: Danielle Di Michiel
Designed by Mark Latter @ pinkstripedesign.com
Photography by Eddie MacDonald
Copyedited by Hilary Boddie
Production by Sha Huxtable
Models: Victoria Hodgson, Delphine Gaborit,
Raquel Meseguer, Patrick McErlean and Moeen Latif

DISCLAIMER The author and publisher cannot accept any
responsibility for misadventure resulting from the practice of any
of the techniques or principles in this book. It is not intended to be
and should not be used as guidance for the treatment of serious
health problems; please refer to a medical professional if you have
concerns about any aspect of your condition or fitness level.

ACKNOWLEDGEMENTS

I owe so much thanks to so many colleagues and friends that it is
almost impossible to pick out a few names.

Danielle Di Michiel at Kyle Cathie, thank you so much for your expert
guiding hand which has helped bring this book to publication.

Eddie MacDonald, our photographer, made the shoot enormous fun.
His experienced eye and attention to detail has led me to believe that if
he wanted a change of career, Pilates teaching would be a good choice!
Marie Anne Coultier, thanks for making us look great. Moeen, Delphine,
Raquel, Patrick and Helen – you were a delight to work with – thank you.

Kate Fernyhough, Chartered Physiotherapist and Body Control Pilates
teacher. I have been fortunate to work closely with Kate now for several
years. She has been gracious enough to read through this manuscript
and to offer her advice, so thank you Kate for your wisdom and in particular
for pointing out that 150 hours of Pilates per week might be a bit excessive
(I'd meant 150 minutes!). Kate has a well established Private Practice in
Staffordshire and can be contacted at eccleshall.physio@fsmail.net

The knowledge within this book and the inspiration for many of the
exercises comes from the collective work of an amazing team of
Body Control Pilates teachers. I must particularly thank Lisa Bradshaw,
Nathan Gardner, Sarah Marks and all our studio staff for their creativity
and technical skills. I am both incredibly proud of them and incredibly
grateful to them.

Bridget Montague, whose gentle patience when teaching me has helped
me to understand my body so well. Thank you! And last, but by no means
least, Victoria Hodgson, a member of our teacher training team, part-time
model (she graces many of the pages of this book) and fantastic friend.
This book would not have been written or published without you!

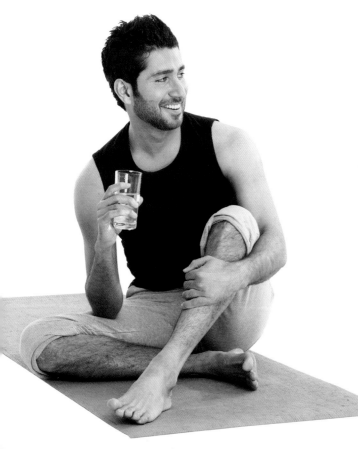

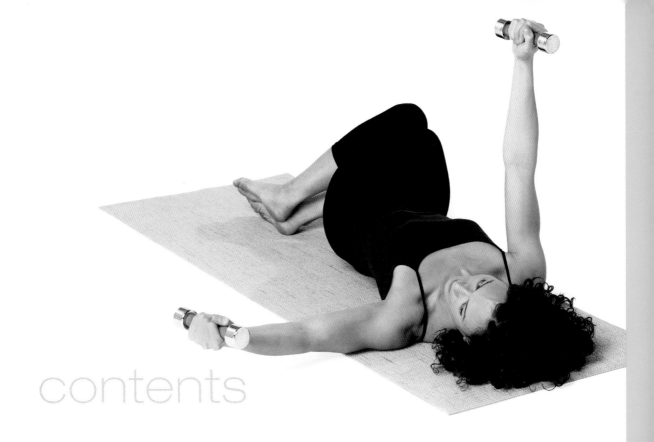

contents

introduction

'In 10 sessions you'll feel the difference, in 20 you'll see the difference,
in 30 you'll have a whole new body.'

JOSEPH PILATES, *RETURN TO LIFE THROUGH CONTROLOGY.*

And what a body you'll have!

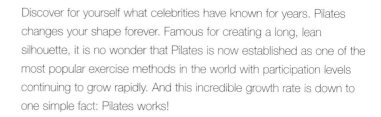

Discover for yourself what celebrities have known for years. Pilates changes your shape forever. Famous for creating a long, lean silhouette, it is no wonder that Pilates is now established as one of the most popular exercise methods in the world with participation levels continuing to grow rapidly. And this incredible growth rate is down to one simple fact: Pilates works!

But is Pilates a good choice for long-term weight loss?

The answer is a resounding 'yes', because Pilates involves strength training, which is crucial for successfully losing weight and, most importantly, for keeping it off. By strength training, we do not mean heavy bodybuilding. Don't worry, you will not bulk up with Pilates, but you will be able to sculpt and create the body you want.

Let's look at some of the myths about weight loss and find out why Pilates as strength training is so effective. Perhaps a good starting point is to clarify what we really want to achieve. Do we really want to lose weight or do we really mean that we want to lose body fat? The problem with just looking at the scales is that you may be losing muscle alongside fat. You will start to lose weight when the energy (calories) that you use is more than the energy that you consume.

So it should be a simple equation of 'do more, eat less'. But many of you who've tried this formula will know that it's not that simple. People try to starve themselves to lose weight, thinking that it is all about counting calories. But reducing calorie intake is just part of the solution. What matters most is making your body more efficient at burning calories. That is, improving your metabolic rate. To do this you need to create lean body mass, because this is the muscle mass underneath your body fat which burns calories day in, day out even when you are resting!

For a weight-loss programme to be successful long-term, you will need to have the right muscle mass to maintain this high metabolic rate. Yes, if you starve yourself, you may lose body fat and weigh less on the scales, but without a strength training routine like Pilates you will also lose the muscle resources you need to keep your metabolic rate high. In fact, your metabolic rate may actually slow down and you may not be able to maintain the weight loss because every time you eat a few extra calories you will pile back on the pounds.

Now, all types of exercise will burn calories and develop muscle tissue. Where Pilates excels is in its ability to build lean muscle tissue, thus enabling your body to be more efficient at burning calories even when you have finished your workout and are going about your normal activities. Furthermore, the Pilates exercises in this book have been chosen especially for their muscle-building effects. Many have been modified to increase their efficiency for toning muscles. The workouts include weight-bearing exercises which use the body's own weight against gravity, free weights and resistance to help you build more muscle and lose fat. This makes Pilates one of the best ways to control your weight in both the short- and long-term, avoiding the typical 'yo yo effect' of your weight going up and down.

How does this Pilates for Weight Loss programme differ from a normal Pilates workout? The exercises in this book have been modified to heighten their body-toning effects. Where applicable, exercises have been combined to enable you to 'double' the benefits, for example Ribcage Closure with Leg Slide (page 49), Hip Rolls with a Single Arm Fly (page 69) and Dart into Side Bend (page 105).

This total body-conditioning regime will enable you to sculpt your body the way you want it. While the whole body (and mind) is involved in every Pilates exercise, the precision with which you perform the movements will enable you to focus on specific areas. You will be able to 'chisel' your body into shape!

To maximise your weight loss and to help you achieve optimal health and well-being, we have also included chapters on cross-training with cardiovascular activities, eating well and making positive lifestyle choices.

the pilates story

joseph pilates' legacy

The exercises in this book are based on the work of Joseph Pilates. Born in Germany in 1883, he was, to use a well-worn cliché, years ahead of his time. The importance he intuitively placed on fundamentals, such as core strength, would come to be clinically recognised in research studies carried out more than twenty years after his death.

Incorporating elements drawn from martial arts, body-building and yoga, Joseph first developed a series of matwork exercises, and then, while interned in Lancaster after the outbreak of the First World War, he devised equipment, using even bed springs and leather straps so that bedridden internees could still exercise their limbs.

Yet it was really out of the New York studio that he set up with his wife, Clara, in the late 1920s, that the Pilates Method was defined. For Joe and Clara, it was a way of life rather than a business. While his first clients were mostly from the boxing community, the proximity of the New York City Ballet encouraged dancers to seek out Joe when they were injured. After his death, Clara continued to run the studio for as long as she was able before handing on the baton to some of the teachers who had worked with Joseph in his studio. Each of these teachers developed the Method in their own way, thereby giving birth to the different approaches to the Pilates Method that we see today.

the body control pilates story

There are many different reasons why people take up Pilates. For me, it was pain from a herniated disc that persuaded me that I had to try this, then little heard of, exercise method. Pilates had an immediate and positive impact on my back problem. I hadn't started classes with a view to losing weight, but was very pleasantly surprised when I did! In fact, I was so impressed by the changes to my body and body awareness that I decided to teach Pilates rather than history!

After completing my training in London, I began to realise that although Joseph Pilates had left us an amazing legacy of work, many of his original exercises were simply too challenging for the average body. I think it helped my understanding that my own body was decidedly average. With this in mind, we started to break Joseph's exercises down, modifying them, taking on board recent medical research and developing a very specific approach, which we called Body Control Pilates. Many of the exercises in our programme are unique to Body Control Pilates. Our goal has always been to make Pilates as accessible as possible for the average person, irrespective of age and fitness level. We have succeeded in this and the Body Control Pilates Association has become Europe's largest professional body for Pilates teachers.

optimum health and well-being

There are so many reasons why people begin Pilates: managing back problems, preventing injuries, greater flexibility, stress management or simply to shape up flabby buttocks and flatten stomachs.

Whatever the reasons for initially starting classes, I can guarantee that the reason people continue is because it makes them feel great. The health benefits include:

Improved posture and body use Pain in joints and muscles is usually down to poor body use and posture. It is the tissues of the muscles and the joints which suffer when we lack awareness of good posture and optimum body use.

Improved circulation, joint mobility and healing Pilates works on the concept that the body has the potential to heal itself. Its movements work at a cellular level to channel the blood flow to all regions of the body, carrying nutrients and taking away toxins.

Improved bone density As a strength-training method, Pilates can help to build up your bone bank. The stronger your muscles are, the greater the tug on the bones which in turn helps to stimulate bone growth.

Stress relief An understanding of the movements in Pilates, deep breathing and release of tension, combine to bring a sense of calm and relaxation.

A better immune system Studies have shown that regular exercise helps to boost the immune system. Joseph Pilates was proud that none of the regulars who attended his daily exercise class at the internment camp died from the terrible Spanish flu epidemic.

An enhanced sex life Pilates can help your sex life by improving your body awareness, your self confidence and self esteem, your flexibility and last, but by no means least, it can help to strengthen the pelvic floor muscles.

Improved balance and co-ordination As we age, these skills may make all the difference to our quality of life. Pilates can help to reduce your risk of falling and fracturing bones.

Anti-ageing benefits Pilates can help to give you a body that is both strong and supple, right through your later years, but it can also help to keep your skin supple too. Collagen gives your skin its elasticity but is slow to regenerate. To help keep your skin's youthful elasticity, you need to do exercises which stretch it as this maximises the production of DHEA (dehydroepiandrosterone) which is responsible for protecting collagen. Two hours of stretching per week, combined with cardio activities are recommended. This keeps your joints naturally lubricated, and new research shows that exercise actually changes the lubricating fluid so that it contains more of the chemicals that restore collagen.

posture perfect

The new you is going to start right now. I want you to stop and think about how you are sitting or standing as you read this book. I suspect that as you read those words you began to make some subtle changes to your posture. Perhaps you sat up a bit, you might even have pulled your stomach in? I think most of us know how we should be sitting it's just that as we go about our daily activities, we forget. This is a shame, as there is no quicker fix to improve your appearance than by sitting or standing tall.

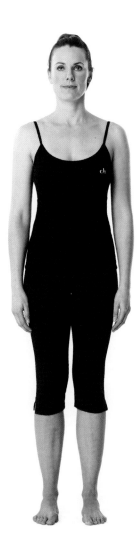

Stand in front of a mirror in your underwear. Now slouch. I can guarantee that it will not be a pretty sight. Poor posture means you appear shorter, your stomach sticks out, your pectorals (if you are male) disappear, your breasts (if you are female) look saggy and your waist disappears as your ribs sink toward your hips.

Now try the same experiment but this time stand tall. Elongate your spine by lengthening up through the crown of your head. Open your shoulders, allowing your arms to relax down by your sides. Gently draw your lower abdominals back towards your spine (more on this later in the book). Breathe. Observe the changes. You will instantly look taller, your breasts will be lifted, your waist has reappeared and your stomach will look flatter.

The problem is that for most of us standing tall is very tiring. It requires activity from the deep postural muscles to keep upright. Your deep 'core' muscles are basically anti-gravity muscles. When they are weak, it is very difficult to maintain good posture. Pilates can give you this core strength from within, the ability to stand tall easily day in, day out. This is what has drawn performers to Pilates for years. It will give you that natural grace and elegance, or 'graceful carriage', as Joseph Pilates called it.

Posture and movement are inseparable; it is, in fact, impossible to stand still. We may think that we are standing still but in fact our muscles and our nerves are making hundreds of tiny adjustments in response to the pull of gravity and our surroundings. Our habitual posture and how we move are affected by a wide variety of influences ranging from genetics to personal and medical history, environmental and cultural influences. To facilitate any lasting changes, you will need to understand and experience how to use your body well. This is what you will be doing when you practise the Pilates exercises in this book. Alongside helping to build lean muscle tissue and reshaping your body, you will also be learning good body use as you experience good posture and movement.

the problem of obesity

Being overweight, obese or morbidly obese significantly increases the risk of developing many diseases such as diabetes, hypertension, heart disease, strokes and osteoarthritis.

A 2006 survey, published by the National Health Service, found that in 2005, 23.1 per cent of men in England were obese, compared to 13.2 per cent in 1993. A similar trend is evident amongst English women with 24.8 per cent classified as obese in 2005, compared to 16.4 per cent in 1993. Perhaps more worryingly, in 2005 about one child in six, aged between two and ten years old, could be considered obese. An individual is considered obese when their Body Mass Index (BMI) measures 30 or higher (see page 13), and morbidly obese when they weigh more than 100 pounds over their ideal body weight or have a BMI of 40 or higher.

How these figures have got so high is a matter of concern, as the problem is, in principle, easy to identify and solve. The adoption of healthy eating habits is central to solving the problem, as is the development of a healthy and active lifestyle. If you think you may be obese or if you feel that have a lot of weight to lose, please contact your local GP who can offer you advice and support.

Can Pilates help you? I believe the answer is yes. If you are seriously overweight, you are often caught in a Catch-22 scenario. Around 50 per cent of adults say that their health is not good enough to partake in active sports or physical activity and yet it is clear that they need exercise to help improve their health and lose weight. I am hoping that, with your doctor's permission, you may be able to try some of the gentle movements in this Pilates programme and also the suggestions for becoming more active in the chapter on cardiovascular activities. The Fundamental exercises (pages 19–47) would be a great starting point.

As you gain more confidence in your ability to move, you will gradually be able to increase your overall levels of activity. Start gently by becoming more active in your everyday life. Remember that every little extra activity will help. You could start simply with walking more. As this becomes easier, you can try walking a little faster for a few minutes and so gradually build up your level of fitness. Regular medical check-ups are essential and combined with the healthy eating and lifestyle advice later in the book, you will be able to reap all the benefits this programme can offer.

how much weight do you want to lose?

Normal bathroom weighing scales can give you a rough idea but they can also distort the truth about how much fat you are carrying. If you only consider your weight in pounds and ounces, then you may get the wrong answer as it is perfectly feasible for someone to be well within their ideal weight range, yet still be carrying too much fat. For example, a very fit muscular person may weigh the same as an unfit plumper person on the scales because muscle is heavier than fat.

A similar confusion may arise if you simply use the scales to measure your progress. As you exercise more, you will shed fat and replace it with muscle tissue. You will feel your body become tauter, firmer and more toned, and your clothes will fit better. You may drop a clothes size, but if you hop on the scales, you may weigh the same as when you started! I am not saying that you should throw away your bathroom scales, as they can give you a rough indicator as to how you are doing, but we are going to need a more accurate way to work out how much you need to lose and also to measure how much progress you are making.

BODY MASS INDEX

Our bodies are made up of two components: lean body mass and fat. Lean body mass consists of organs such as the heart, the liver, the pancreas, bones, skin and, of course, muscle tissue. All of these need oxygen and nutrients from food to grow and repair. Muscle, in particular, has a high metabolic rate and burns calories quickly. Apart from lean body mass, the rest of your body consists of fat. Fat does not need oxygen, does not repair itself and has a low metabolic rate, so it doesn't burn calories.

Some body fat is essential to the body – it keeps us warm and insulated. If you are female and have too little body fat, you may run the risk of decreased fertility associated with amenorrhea (when menstruation ceases). This in turn may have an effect on the long-term health of your bones.

What we need to consider is the ratio of lean body mass to fat. Your lean body mass is constantly altering because of the changes in your muscles. People who have a low lean body mass often lack energy and studies have shown that they are equally at risk from degeneration and premature ageing as people who have too much body fat. This is a very good reason why you should not rely on faddish slimming diets as opposed to exercise and a healthy diet to stay slim. Faddish diets with no exercise will have you losing muscle tissue, resulting in a loss of muscle tone and low energy levels.

The way to streamline your body, improve your energy levels, boost your immune system and achieve optimum health lies in increasing your lean body mass with exercise and a healthy balanced diet.

The most commonly-used method to assess if your weight is putting your health at risk is the Body Mass Index (BMI). This is used by doctors and fitness professionals around the world. The BMI takes into account both your height and your weight. For this, you use a set formula. Although BMI alone doesn't give you information about your body fat, using it in conjunction with waist-to-hip circumference ratio (page 14) will give you a better idea of how much weight you need to lose.

measuring your body mass index (BMI)

BMI = your weight (in kilograms) ÷ your height (in metres) squared.
For example, 60kg ÷ (1.65m x 1.65m) = 22

results

Below 18.5: Underweight. This means that you may need to gain weight for your health's sake. Please consult your doctor if you have any concerns or if you feel afraid to put on weight.

18.5–25: Normal. This does not mean that you cannot lose some weight for appearance's sake, but for your health you should stay in this range. Remember, though, that you may still need to tone up.

25–30: Overweight. You should lose some weight for your health's sake.

30–40: Obese. Your health is at risk. Losing weight will improve your health.

Over 40: Morbidly obese. You should visit your doctor for a health check before you try any exercise.

Unfortunately, the BMI is still not the full picture. A pound of muscle tissue weighs the same as a pound of fat, but muscle tissue takes up less space than fat, which is why the guy with the six pack might weigh the same as the guy with the beer belly – but six pack guy's jeans fit better! It is also not accurate during pregnancy, if you are breastfeeding or if you are very frail.

WAIST-TO-HIP RATIO

This measurement divides the circumference of your waist by the circumference of your hips. This is a very important measurement as we know that the distribution of fat in the body has considerable health implications. Fat which is stored around the waist has been shown to be linked with health problems, particularly an increased risk of non-insulin diabetes, heart disease, high blood pressure and abnormal blood fat levels. In women, this 'central obesity', which creates a typical apple-shape figure, is associated with a higher risk of pre-menopausal breast cancer. Fat stored around the hips creating a typical 'pear shape' seems to be less problematic.

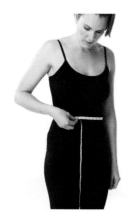

measuring your waist-to-hip ratio

1. Waist
Stand tall, but relax your waist (no zipping or hollowing – that's cheating). Locate the narrowest point of your waist (normally around the navel) and measure there.

2. Hip
Still standing tall, find the widest point of your hips and buttocks and measure this.

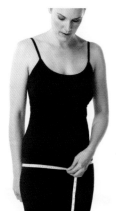

3. Waist-to-hip ratio
Divide the results from 1 (waist) by the results from 2 (hip). This would be your waist-to-hip ratio.

reading the scores
If you are female, you should aim for a waist-to-hip ratio of less than 0.80.
If you are male, you should aim for a waist-to-hip ratio of less than 0.90.

HEALTHY WEIGHT LOSS

Before you begin this weight-loss programme, work out your BMI as above and your waist-to-hip ratio. Work out how much weight you wish to lose. Bear in mind that health professionals encourage you to aim for a weight loss of 5–10 per cent over a three to six month period. How does this translate? Well, let's say that you weigh 80kg; a healthy weight loss over six months would be around 8kg. Your goal weight would be 72kg.

The ideal rate of weight loss to aim for to remain healthy is 1–2lbs (0.5–1 kg) per week. This may sound very slow, but bear in mind that we are aiming for healthy weight loss and optimum health. Although you may only be losing 1–2lbs per week, your body shape will be changing noticeably. You will be losing inches! Your body will be more toned and streamlined.

If your BMI score classified you as overweight then your goal will be to bring your score into the 'normal' acceptable categories. Similarly, if your waist-to-hip ratio was over the norm, then your goal will be to bring the ratio back within the recommended guidelines.

To help you keep a record of your progress and to help to establish the best ways to achieve your goals, you may like to complete this plan.

personal weight-loss plan

Date

Current weight

Height

Body mass index (BMI)

Waist measurement

Hip measurement

Waist-to-hip ratio

How wuch weight do you wish to lose over the

next six months?

How many steps do you take each day?

(if you have a pedometer)

When are the best times for you to do your 150 minutes of

Pilates practice?

When are the best times and days for you to do your

150 minutes of cardiovascular activities (see page 138)?

How are you going to monitor your progress?

How are you going to reward yourself for progress made?

how to get the most out of the programme

Ideally you would read through all the chapters of the book, except the exercises themselves, before starting the programme. In the meantime, this is a very simple guide to how to use this book.

1. Read Before You Begin (opposite) and make sure you have all the right equipment.
2. Weigh yourself on accurate scales, naked or in your underwear, first thing in the morning.
3. Work out your Body Mass Index (page 13) and work out your Waist-to-Hip Ratio (page 14). Add this to your Personal Weight-Loss Plan (page 15).
4. Read the chapter on how to maximise your weight loss by cross-training, eating well, and making lifestyle changes (pages 138–157).
5. Consult with your doctor/medical practitioner and complete the rest of the Personal Weight-Loss Plan, taking into account your doctor's advice. Set your goals.
6. Read the chapter on Fundamentals (page 18), then practise the exercises until perfect!
7. Start the All Levels workouts (pages 108–111). Read through and learn all the exercises listed in the workouts before you try them. Gradually work up to 150 minutes of Pilates practice per week.
8. Include a Sculpting Workout (pages 124–129) if you wish, for any problem areas.
9. Start to become more active by increasing the amount of incidental exercise that you do, e.g. increase the number of steps you take each day. Record these in your Training Diary (page 139).
10. Work out your target heart rate (page 141) and record this in your Training Diary (page 139).
11. Plan your cardiovascular activities for each week (pages 138–143). Aim for 150 minutes per week. Record your cardiovascular activities in your Training Diary (page 139).
12. Clear your kitchen cupboards and fridge of any unhealthy processed food and stock up on healthier foods (see pages 144–150).
13. Plan some relaxation time into your schedule and ensure that you are getting enough sleep.
14. Every two weeks, weigh yourself on the same scales at the same time wearing the same underwear (washed of course!). Record the results. Similarly, work out your BMI and waist-to-hip ratio again and compare results.
15. Record your progress, goals achieved and reward yourself as appropriate! If you are not making progress, try to establish why and address the problem.
16. Re-assess your Pilates and cardiovascular level of ability at regular intervals. Look out for signs that you are ready to move up a level of difficulty.
17. Consider adding variety to your workouts by following the advice given on pages 154–156.

before you begin

Here is a list of the equipment you are going to need for your Pilates practice.

A padded non-slip mat or a yoga mat folded in half.

A folded towel or small flat pillow.

A plump pillow.

A stretch band of medium strength or a long stretchy scarf.

Hand-held weights of 0.5kg–4kg (approximately 1–10lbs) each.

Ankle weights of 0.5kg–1kg (approximately 1–2.5lbs) for each
    weight. Some weights allow you to adjust the weight in
    increments.

A notebook to use as your Training Diary.

A tape measure to calculate your waist-to-hip ratio and a set of
    bathroom scales (not pictured).

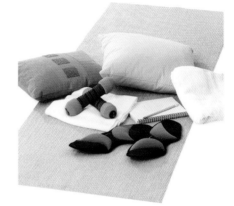

You can make your own ankle weights with a pair or stockings
(or by cutting the tops off tights). Weigh out 500g of rice or lentils,
or more as you progress. Tie a knot in the leg about 15cm from the foot. Fill the tights with the rice
and tie another knot. You can then wrap the homemade weight around your ankle. Similarly, you
can use a can of beans or a small bottle of water as a hand weight. You will need to be careful of
your wrist alignment if you do this, as the grip will be different to commercial weights. Make sure
that your wrist isn't being held at an awkward angle.

BEFORE YOU START A WORKOUT

Prepare the space by making it warm, comfortable and free from distractions. Make sure that you
have enough room to move your arms and legs freely. If you like, you can play some background
music, but it should be quiet and not distracting.

Do not exercise if you are feeling unwell, have been drinking alcohol or have just eaten a heavy
meal. Similarly, avoid exercise if you have an injury or are undergoing medical treatment or taking
medication.

Remember, it is always wise to consult your doctor before taking up a new exercise regime. For
example, many of the exercises are wonderful for back-related problems, but you should always
seek expert guidance first. Similarly, not all the exercises in this programme are suitable for use
during pregnancy.

fundamentals

The following pages are, without question, the most important pages in the book. Imagine that this is a cookery book and the exercises are the recipes. This section would be all about cookery skills; how to boil, steam, fry and roast along with the list of all the raw ingredients you are going to need. Without these skills and without the right ingredients, even the best recipe will fail.

Whatever your level of fitness or Pilates experience, you should still revisit these fundamental exercises on a regular basis. Our method is constantly evolving, taking on board new scientific research. Wherever applicable, we incorporate these new approaches and ideas into our teaching. In this book, I have introduced some new techniques for learning core stability with the Variable Zip (see page 27). These are only subtle changes, but I hope you find them useful.

Body Control Pilates has built its world-wide reputation on its unique approach to the teaching of the fundamentals of Pilates. In our minds, this is where you succeed or fail in your practice. If the basics are not right, then your practice of the exercises will be flawed and this programme will not deliver its promises. In an ideal world, you would be attending classes with a qualified teacher to help you to understand these basics. In the absence of a teacher, however, you have the exercises in this section. Practise them diligently. They will help you to understand your body and its movements. The three areas we will be focusing on in this section are how to find good postural alignment in a variety of positions, how to breathe efficiently during the exercises and how to improve your core stability. The order in which I have presented the basic exercises follows the order in which I would normally teach a new client.

Eight principles underlie every movement in our approach to exercise:

1. Relaxation
2. Concentration
3. Alignment
4. Breathing

5. Centring – core strength
6. Co-ordination
7. Flowing movements
8. Stamina

With each and every exercise, it is vital that you are aware of how you are moving. Pilates has been called 'intelligent exercise' not because you need brains to perform the exercises but because you need to 'think' about what you are doing. Pilates is both mind and body training. I believe that Joseph Pilates drew his inspiration from the martial arts of the Far East – slow, controlled, flowing movements performed with thoughtful awareness. He taught that one of the main results of his method was gaining the mastery of your mind over the complete control of your body. Even when the exercises become familiar to you, you must still use your mind to control your body. By adding new challenges to your routines, you will be able to progress to the advanced work.

standing tall

Have you ever thought just how difficult it is to stand tall for any length of time? Usually what happens after a few minutes is that we start to shift our weight around from one leg onto the other. We start to droop and sag. Most people do not have enough activity in their deep postural muscles to maintain good posture for any length of time. This is what Pilates can teach you.

AIM

To promote awareness of good posture.

Starting Position

Stand on the floor, not on the mat. Place your feet hip-width apart in a natural stance – that is, neither turned out nor in a rigid, parallel position. Have your arms relaxed and down by your sides.

'Standing is also very important and should be practised at all times until it is mastered' JOSEPH PILATES, *RETURN TO LIFE THROUGH CONTROLOGY*

ACTION

1. Sway forwards slightly from the ankle joint so that you feel your weight shift onto the balls of the foot and the toes. Keep your heels down.

2. Sway backwards through centre so that you feel your weight shift onto the heels. Keep the toes on the floor.

3. Sway back to centre and become aware of the three points of your feet – the base of the big toe, the base of the small toe and the centre of the heel. This forms a triangle. Feel your weight centred on this triangle.

4. Gently lock your knees back, then release them. The idea is that they should be straight but not locked.

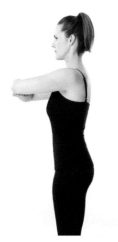

5. Bring your awareness to your pelvis now. Gently tilt the pelvis forward, your pubic bone will move backwards (see photo left).

6. Now gently tilt the pelvis backwards into a posterior tilt, your pubic bone will move forward (see photo top right).

7. Now place your pelvis in the mid-neutral position (we will be working more on finding neutral on page 24).

8. Without moving the tailbone, feel it lengthening down towards the floor. Your hips should feel open.

9. Now lift your waist up and away from your pelvis, feeling your deep abdominals work as you do this.

10. Become aware of your ribcage and your natural breathing.

11. Feel your shoulder-blades widening across your back whilst your collarbones widen across the front of your shoulders.

12. Allow your arms to hang free and easy from your shoulders.

13. Lengthen up through the crown of the head, releasing your neck and allowing your head to balance freely on top of the spine.

14. Focus forwards, softening your gaze.

15. Become aware of a sense of opposition through the body. As you lengthen upwards through your spine, you also lengthen the tailbone downwards. Ground yourself through the two triangles of the feet.

16. Breathe!

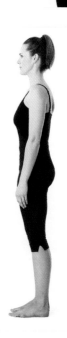

breathing

Just why is breathing so important to practising Pilates? If you have ever tried a meditation class, you will know that one of the first things the teacher will get you to do is to focus on your breathing. There is no better way to bring your mind into the moment. If you are focusing on your breathing, you are thinking about your body now, at this moment in time. Furthermore, breathing is directly related to the body's skeletal alignment. Nearly all the muscles involved in the breathing process also have a postural function. So, posture, breathing and movement are closely interrelated. What we need to do is learn how to improve the efficiency of our breathing, which will help to increase your oxygen intake. This is vital while exercising and a skill to last a lifetime.

Stand in front of a mirror and watch as you take a deep breath. Do your shoulders rise up around the ears or perhaps your lower stomach expands when you breathe in? None of this is wrong, but we may be able to improve it. We want your lungs to expand in all directions like a balloon. The problem is that many of us only partially inflate the balloon and do not fully deflate it either. If you completely exhale, you will naturally stimulate a deeper inhalation.

Joseph Pilates taught his clients to squeeze every atom of air from their lungs until they were almost as free of air as a vacuum. In this way, your lungs will automatically completely refill themselves with fresh air.

In order to maximise your breath while doing the exercises, we are going to use lateral thoracic breathing, which involves breathing wide and full into your ribcage. This makes sense as the lungs are situated in the ribcage – by expanding it, the volume of the cavity is increased and the capacity for oxygen intake is therefore also increased. It also encourages maximum use of the lower part of the lungs.

This type of breathing makes the upper body more fluid and mobile. The lungs become like bellows, with the lower ribcage expanding wide as you breathe in and then closing down as you breathe out. Now, as you breathe in your diaphragm will automatically descend. The aim is not to stop this but, rather, to focus on the movement to be widthways and into the back. This will also be helpful when you need to use your abdominals to stabilise.

ACTION

Try this simple breathing exercise

1. Sit or stand tall. Wrap a stretch band, scarf or towel around your ribs, crossing it over at the front.

2. Holding the opposite ends of the scarf and gently pulling it tight, breathe in and allow your ribs to expand the scarf (watch that you do not lift the breastbone too high).

3. As you breathe out, you may gently squeeze the scarf or stretch band to help to fully empty your lungs and relax the ribcage, allowing the breastbone to soften.

Practise this a little and often. Take care not to 'over breathe'. If you start to feel light-headed or dizzy, stop and try again later.

Throughout the exercises in this book, you will find directions on when exactly to breathe in and when to breathe out as you perform the exercise. Learning this is part of the mind-body challenge. Each exercise has its own breathing pattern which has been chosen to help facilitate the movements. The most common pattern is to:

– Breathe in to prepare for a movement
– Breathe out, stabilise (zip) and move
– Breathe in, still zipped, to recover

If you do get confused, don't stop breathing! Never hold your breath.

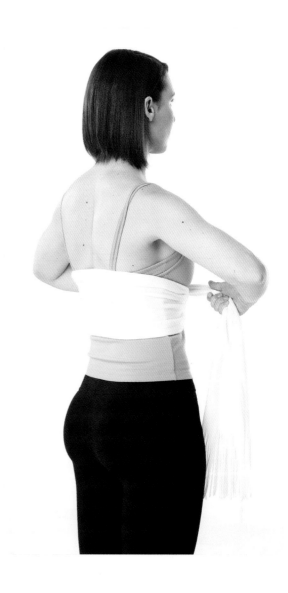

the relaxation position

The Relaxation Position is both an exercise and the start and finish position for many of the lying exercises. As such, it is probably one of the most important positions to get right.

The Relaxation Position can be used to release unwanted tension and improve body awareness of good postural alignment, breathing, and stability. As a starting position, use it to check your alignment, breathing and stability.

Starting Position

Lie on your back on the mat with your knees bent, feet hip-width apart and in parallel. If you aim your heels towards the centre of each buttock, you'll be about hip-width apart.

ACTION

If you need to, place a small folded towel or firm, flat pillow underneath the head. The idea is for your neck to be lengthened but to maintain its natural, cervical curve. The head should be neither tipped forward nor back. Sometimes a pillow is not necessary, or you may need a couple.

If you are going to remain in the Relaxation Position, place your hands on the lower abdomen to allow the shoulders to widen and open. If you are using the Relaxation Position as a starting position, have your arms relaxed down by your sides, palms facing the floor.

Watchpoints

- Do not 'collapse' in this position. Stay aware of your body.
- Notice which parts of the body are in touch with the mat.
- Feel the three areas of body weight: your head, the sacrum at the back of the pelvis and your ribcage. Allow the floor to support them.
- Allow your spine to release and lengthen.
- Become aware of the triangle on the soles of each foot (see point 3, page 19).
- Soften your neck, your jaw and your gaze.
- Think wide and open across your collarbones.
- Allow time for the body to adapt to this position and allow the spine to release.
- Notice any areas of tension and allow them to melt gently into the floor.

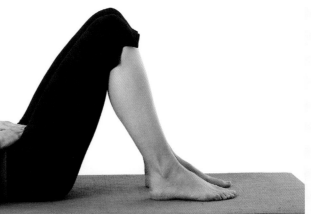

finding neutral in the relaxation position (the compass)

For resting positions and for many of the exercises, you will be asked to find and/or keep your natural, neutral pelvic and spinal positions. The angle of your pelvis will affect the angle of your spine. Learning how to find your neutral pelvis is the first step towards finding your neutral spinal position.

Starting Position

The Relaxation Position. Imagine you have a compass on your lower abdomen. The navel is north and the pubic bone south, with west and east on either side. We are going to look at two incorrect positions in order to find the correct one.

ACTION

1. Tilt your pelvis to the north, that is towards your navel (see photo below). The pelvis will tuck under, the waist will flatten and the curve of the lower back is lost as your tailbone lifts off the mat. You will also grip the muscles around your hips and abdominals.

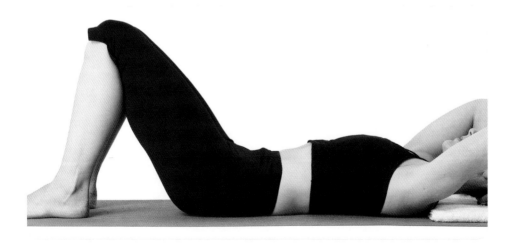

2. Next, carefully and gently move the pelvis in the other direction so that it tilts south (avoid this bit if you have a back injury). The lower back will arch, the ribs flare and the stomach sticks out (see photo right). Gently roll back to the Starting Position.

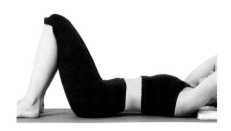

3. Your neutral pelvic position is midway between these two extremes. Go back to the image of the compass and think of the pointer as a spirit level. When you are in neutral, the pubic bone and pelvic bones will be level North, South, East and West. Your sacrum will rest squarely on the mat. You should feel as though the tailbone is lengthening away along the mat. Try also to keep both sides of the waist long and equal.

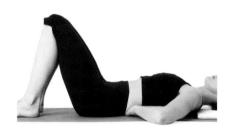

4. Now bring your awareness to your spine. Think of the long 'S' shape of the spine, lengthen through the spine while keeping those natural curves. Normally, you should still have a gentle curve in your neck and a gentle curve in the lumbar spine. You should be able to just slip the back of your hand under your waist. Now bring your awareness back to allow the weight of the head, the ribcage and the back of the pelvis to sink into the mat.

BREATHING IN THE RELAXATION POSITION

Follow directions 1–4 above.

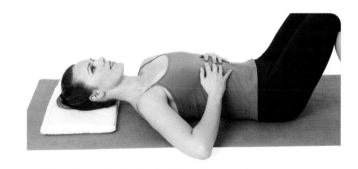

5. Place your hands onto your ribcage. Breathe in wide and full to the back and sides of your ribcage. Feel your fingers separate as you do so.

6. Breathe out fully and completely, allowing the ribcage to close naturally as you do so.

7. Feel the in-breath come in spontaneously, directing it as above.

Watchpoints

- Think wide and open across your shoulders.
- Do not over-breathe.
- Stop if you feel light-headed.

pilates core strength – centring

Now that you have learnt how to recognise good postural alignment and are familiar with lateral thoracic breathing, it is time to learn about centring or what is often referred to as 'core stability'.

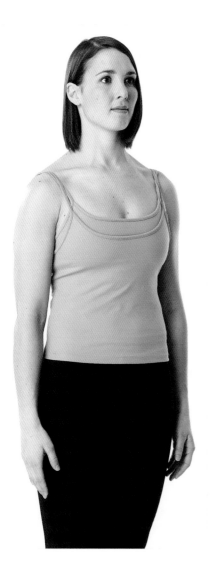

Pilates-style 'centring' is probably best explained as the ability to control your movements from the centre or core outwards. Why do we do this? Well, if you can imagine doing an exercise like Scissors on page 67 without core control, your pelvis would move as your legs lower; this might then cause your back to arch and you could potentially damage your back. Similarly, with the same exercise, without good scapular and cervical stability, you risk injury to your neck and shoulders.

The idea is to utilise the deep abdominals, which wrap around you like a corset, together with the deep back muscle (multifidus) and the pelvic floor muscles to create a solid protective base that stabilises the spine, supports the back and helps to prevent injury. Creating a strong centre is key if you are going to do the Pilates exercises effectively. Our goal is good, natural movement achieved with economy of effort and no strain.

Think of your 'core' as running down your centre (like an apple core), through your three body weights: the head, ribcage and pelvis.

To help your core stability you are going to learn the following:
– How to keep your lumbar spine stable with 'the variable zip'.
– How to move your limbs freely and independently of your pelvis (pelvic stability).
– Good upper body movement, including scapular stability.
– Good head and neck alignment, including cervical stability.

the variable zip

Joseph Pilates instructed students to keep the abdomen drawn in as far as possible while doing his exercises. Over the years, different schools of Pilates have favoured different 'cues' to help achieve this. However, when teaching group classes or when writing books like this, there needs to be 'one cue to suit all'.

Body Control Pilates introduced the 'zip up and hollow' cue to help new clients discover and connect with their core muscles. This 'zip up and hollow' employs a gentle recruitment of the pelvic floor (the 'zip up') to help initiate the deep core muscles (the 'hollow'). Using the 'zip up', also helps to develop good pelvic floor muscles, essential for preventing incontinence, prolapses, prostate problems and, of course, for enhancing your sex life.

The normal pattern for most exercises is to get into the Starting Position. On your out-breath, prior to movement, engage the zip and use it to control your movement until the exercise is finished.

Finding your pelvic floor 'zip' muscles can be quite a challenge. There are all sorts of methods you can use – it's simply a matter of trying them out and working out which works best for you. Among the best cues are:

– Sucking your thumb while drawing up the pelvic floor.
– Drawing your sitting bones together.
– Imagining slowing down the flow of water.
– For the guys, imagine you are peeing up a wall (do not move your back: that's cheating)
  or lift your family jewels.

But my all-time favourite, and the cue I use most with my clients, is what they have nicknamed the 'Wind Zip.' For this, I must thank chartered physiotherapist, Ruth Jones, for her inspiring work.

the wind zip

Starting Position

Sit tall on a sturdy chair. Make sure that your weight is even on both sitting bones and that your spine retains its natural curves.

ACTION

1. Breathe in wide to your ribcage.

Watchpoints

- Do not zip too hard (see below).
- Try to keep your buttock muscles relaxed.
- Keep your neck and jaw relaxed.
- Keep breathing. Try to feel your ribcage moving as it is a sign that you haven't over-engaged.
- If you lose the zip, relax and start again from back to front and up inside.
- Keep the pelvis and spine in neutral.

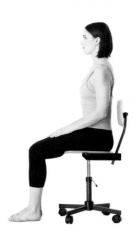

2. Breathe out and imagine that you are about to pass wind. Gently squeeze your back passage (anus) as if trying to prevent passing wind and then bring this feeling forward to your pubic bone. Then gently draw these muscles up inside. You should feel the lower part of your abdominals automatically hollow.

3. Gently hold this zip and breathe normally for five breaths before releasing.

If you find the Wind Zip too difficult, please use our normal zip described in the Pelvic Elevator (opposite) and then gently hollow the lower abdominals. Or you can forget about the pelvic floor and simply scoop the lower abdominals, drawing them back towards the spine. What matters is that you are in control of your body as you move to avoid injury. This will become automatic as you practise more.

how much zip?

One of the most important aspects in all stability work is engaging the muscles at the right amount. Muscles can work from 0–100 per cent effort. Try standing up and tightening your buttocks as much as you can (100 per cent). Now try to release them about 50 per cent. Then let go half that again to 25 per cent – that's how much you should be working your deep muscles. This is because these muscles have to work for you all day, every day – if you work them harder they will fatigue – they need endurance. The key is to vary the amount of 'zip' you use to control the movement. For basic stability work, you should only need a very gentle zip. Of course, when you are doing an advanced exercise you will need to work a bit harder to stay stable.

A good image to keep in mind is a dimmer switch. Adjusting how strongly you use your zip and abdominals is a little like turning the dial on a dimmer switch up or down. The idea is that you only use as much as you need to control the movement. We are looking for economy of effort. The best example of how this works is the Knee Fold. For the simple Single Knee Fold (page 35), you only need a gentle zip. If you want to fold the second knee for the Double Knee Fold (page 36), then you will need to turn the zip up! What happens when you do this is that all the abdominals work together to keep your pelvis and your spine stable as the legs move.

the pelvic elevator zip (sitting)

If you find the Wind Zip does not suit you, then try the more conventional elevator approach.

AIM
This exercise was created to isolate and engage the deep stabilising muscles.

Starting Position
Sit tall on an upright chair making sure that you are sitting square, with the weight even on both sitting bones. Imagine that your pelvic floor is like the lift in a building and this exercise requires you to take the 'lift' up to different floors of the building.

ACTION
1. Breathe in wide and full to your back and sides then lengthen up through the spine.

2. As you breathe out, draw up the muscles of your pelvic floor, as if you are trying to slow the flow of water. Take the pelvic 'lift' up to the first floor of the building. This is as far as you need to engage the muscles for zip and hollow.

3. Breathe in and release the 'lift' back to the ground floor.

It is useful to feel what it is like to pull up the pelvic floor further, so:
4. Breathe out and now take the lift up to the second floor of the building.

5. Breathe in and release.

6. Breathe out and take the lift up to the third floor. Notice how when you do this, all your abdominals engage. Breath in (notice how hard it is to breathe easily). Breathe out and relax.

Watchpoints
- When you reached the first floor, you should have felt the deep lower abdominals engage.
- Do not allow the buttock muscles to join in.
- Keep your jaw relaxed.
- Don't take your shoulders up to the top floor too – keep them down and relaxed.
- Try not to grip around your hips.
- Keep the pelvis and spine quite still.

good alignment and stability on all fours

This is a tricky position to get right as you do not have the floor for feedback. It is the starting position for Table Top (page 73), Leg Pull Front Preparation (page 76) and Leg Pull Front with Push Ups (page 77). To help find the right alignment, study the photo below and look in particular at where the pole touches the head, ribcage and pelvis and where the spine gently curves away from the pole.

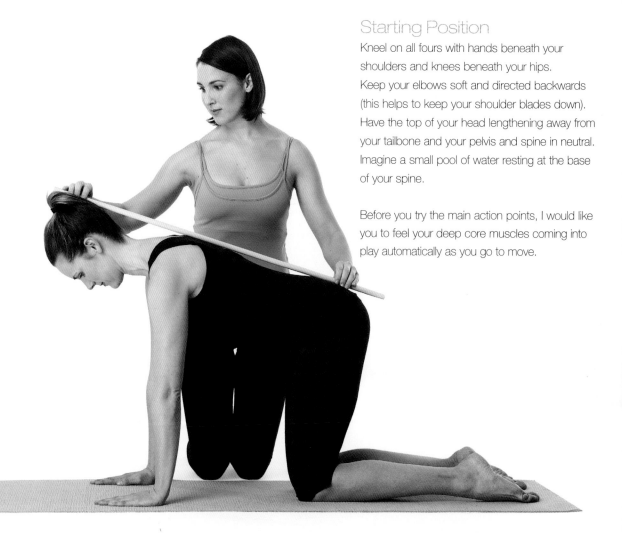

Starting Position

Kneel on all fours with hands beneath your shoulders and knees beneath your hips.
Keep your elbows soft and directed backwards (this helps to keep your shoulder blades down). Have the top of your head lengthening away from your tailbone and your pelvis and spine in neutral. Imagine a small pool of water resting at the base of your spine.

Before you try the main action points, I would like you to feel your deep core muscles coming into play automatically as you go to move.

From this four-point kneeling position, bring your awareness to your trunk. Do not zip or hollow but go to lift one hand from the floor. Can you feel your abdominals automatically engage as you do so? You should be able to feel them wrap around your trunk naturally. These are the very same muscles that we will be strengthening.

ACTION

1. Breathe in wide to prepare.

2. Breathe out and gently zip. Staying zipped throughout, tuck your pelvis under (to compass point 'north' – see page 24), your pubic bone moves forward. The pool of water would roll off your tailbone.

3. Breathe in.

4. Breathe out and tilt the pelvis the other way (to compass point 'south' – take care if you have a back injury). Your tailbone will stick out, the imaginary pool of water would roll up towards your waist.

5. Breathe in.

6. Breathe out and tilt back to find your mid-neutral position. Your pelvic bones and pubic bone are level with the floor. The pool of water stays nestling in the small of your back.

7. Breathe laterally, still zipping gently and holding neutral for five breaths, then release.

Repeat twice.

Watchpoints

- Try to tilt 'north' and 'south' equally within your comfort range.
- Watch that you are neither flaring your ribs towards the floor, nor depressing them too much. They should stay naturally integrated with your waist.
- Avoid rounding your upper back but also avoid pinching the shoulder-blades together.
- Maintain the length and natural curve of your neck. Keep your focus soft and down towards the floor.
- Avoid locking out your elbows.
- Keep the weight on the whole of both hands not just the heel of the hands.
- Think wide and open across your collarbones.
- Maintain the length of the whole spine.
- Maintain equal weight on the hands and the knees throughout the exercise.

good alignment and stability in prone lying

Starting Position

Lie face down on a mat in a straight line. Rest your head on your folded hands. Open and relax your shoulders. You may use a small, flat cushion or folded towel under your abdomen if your lower back is uncomfortable. Your legs should be shoulder-distance apart and relaxed.

ACTION

1. Breathe in wide to the ribcage to prepare.

2. Breathe out, zip gently up from the pelvic floor and feel the lower abdominals drawing up and away from the floor.

3. Breathe in and hold the zip as you breathe laterally for five breaths.

Repeat five times before you release.

Watchpoints

- Imagine there is a precious egg just above the pubic bone that must not be crushed.
- Do not tighten the buttocks.
- There should be no movement in the pelvis or the spine.
- Check that your neck and jaw have stayed relaxed.

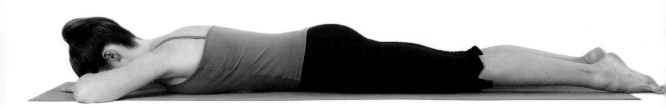

stabilising in the relaxation position

AIM

To feel the difference between a gentle and a strong zip.

Starting Position

Lie in the Relaxation Position.

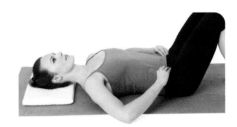

Go through this checklist.

- Is your pelvis in neutral? Your sacrum square on the mat? If not, go through the Compass exercise once more (pages 24–25).
- Be aware of the three main body weights (the head, ribcage and pelvis) sinking into the mat.
- Are your thighs tense or wobbling? You may have to adjust where you place your feet, bringing them nearer to your bottom or taking them further away.
- Become aware of the triangle of the feet, the base of the big toes, the base of the small toes and the centre of the heels.
- Find your hip bones. Place your fingers an inch inwards and downwards from these bones and feel the lower abdominals relaxed.

ACTION

1. Breathe in wide to prepare and lengthen through the spine.

2. Breathe out, gently zip and notice what happens to your lower abdominals. You should be able to feel them engage, gently tensing under your fingers. For a gentle zip, they should stay a bit 'springy'. Do not push into the spine. Keep your tailbone on the floor and lengthen away.

3. Breathe in and release the zip.

4. Breathe out and zip more strongly (as if you've turned up the dial of the dimmer switch). Do not grip any part of your body. You will feel them harden and bulge more.

5. Breathe in and release.

Repeat several times until you can feel the difference.

pelvic stability – leg slides, drops, folds

AIM

Hopefully by now you are confident in how to place your body in good alignment, how to breathe laterally and how to zip. Now it is time to challenge your zip and see if you can control your movements from your core. In the following exercises, you will be learning how to move your limbs whilst keeping the pelvis and spine in neutral.

We will start with small movements then build up to more complicated combinations. Below are four movements to practise, all of them requiring you to keep the pelvis in neutral. A useful image is to imagine that you have a set of car headlamps on your pelvis, shining at the ceiling. The beam should be fixed, not mimicking searchlights! You can vary which exercises you practise in each session, but the Starting Position is the same for all of them.

Starting Position

Lie in the Relaxation Position. Check that your pelvis is in neutral, tailbone down and lengthening away. You may place your hands on your hip bones to check for unwanted movement or leave them down by your sides.

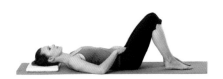

ACTION FOR LEG SLIDES

1. Breathe in wide and full to prepare.

2. Breathe out, zip gently and staying zipped, slide one leg away along the floor in line with your hips. Keep the pelvis stable and in neutral.

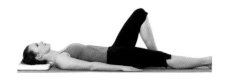

3. Breathe into your lower ribcage while you return the leg to the bent position, trying to keep the bones of the pelvis still.

Watchpoints

- Think of the waist being long and even on both sides as you make the movement.
- Keep your neck and jaw released throughout.
- Avoid tensing or gripping with any part of your body!

- Use a gentle zip to avoid the pelvis tipping.
- Think of drawing the leg back with the back rather than the front of your thigh.
- Keep the foot on the floor and in a line with your hip.

ACTION FOR KNEE OPENINGS

1. Breathe in wide and full to prepare.

2. Breathe out, zip gently and staying zipped, allow one knee to slowly open to the side. Go only as far as allows the pelvis to stay still. It will want to roll side to side – don't let it. How far you can open your knee may depend on the flexibility of your inner thighs and the mobility of your hips.

3. Breathe in, still zipped, as the knee returns to the centre.

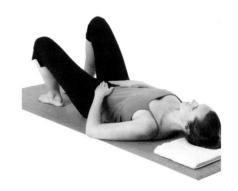

Repeat five times with each leg.

Watchpoints

- Just a gentle zip will keep the pelvis central.
- Keep the other resting leg in line; do not allow it to drop away.
- Feel the weight of your head, ribcage and sacrum (back of pelvis) resting heavily on the mat.

ACTION FOR SINGLE KNEE FOLDS

1. Breathe in wide and full to prepare.

2. Breathe out, zip gently, fold the left knee up. Think of the thighbone dropping down into the hip and anchoring there.

3. Breathe in and hold.

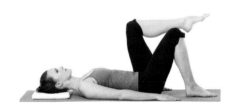

4. Breathe out as you slowly return the foot to the floor.

Repeat five times with each leg.

Watchpoints

- Keep the lower abdominals hollow, don't allow them to bulge.
- Do not rely on the other leg to stabilise you.
- Fold the knee in as far as you can without
- disturbing the pelvis and losing neutral.
- If you find this difficult, try bringing the legs closer to your body.
- Keep the waist equally long on both sides.

ACTION FOR DOUBLE KNEE FOLDS – LEVEL 1

I have put Double Knee Folds here because it is a pelvic stability exercise. Although a fundamental exercise, it is by no means suitable for beginners and should not be attempted until you are very confident with all the other basic exercises in this section. In fact, you may find that you need to practise some of the main programme exercises, for example Oyster (page 78), Table Top (page 73) and Star (page 106), before you try the final version below. In the meantime, I have given you two levels of difficulty.

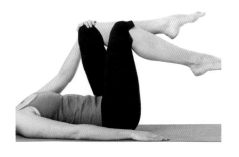

1. Breathe in wide and full to prepare.

2. Breathe out, zip gently and staying zipped, fold one knee up, staying in neutral and keeping the lower abdominals hollow.

3. Breathe in and take hold of the raised knee, with one or both hands.

4. Breathe out, turn your zip up a little and fold the second knee up. Bring the feet together so that the toes are lightly touching, but the knees stay hip-width apart.

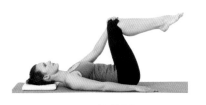

5. Now for the hard bit. Let go of the knee. Breathe in, check that your pelvis is in neutral and that your lower back feels anchored.

6. Breathe out, using the amount of zip you need to keep your back anchored, slowly lower one foot to the floor – do not allow the abdominals to bulge or the pelvis to lose neutral.

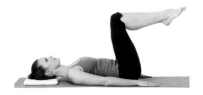

7. Breathe in, then out, unzip a little and slowly lower the other foot.

Repeat six times, alternating which leg you raise and lower first. When you are happy that you can do this version easily, you may raise and lower each leg, still one at a time, but on a single out-breath.

Watchpoints

- You will be surprised by how the body tries to cheat and use everything other than the lower abdominals to stabilise you – be aware of this and keep your neck and shoulders relaxed.

- Make sure your pelvis stays neutral.
- Keep the abdominals hollow.

ACTION FOR DOUBLE KNEE FOLDS – LEVEL 2

Once you are happy with level 1, you can try this.

1. Breathe in wide and full to prepare.

2. Breathe out, zip gently and staying zipped, fold one knee up. Lower abdominals stay hollow. Pelvis neutral.

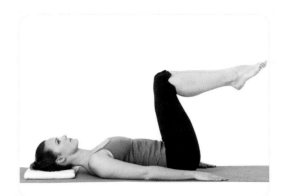

3. Breathe in wide and full.

4. Breathe out and turn up the zip to fold the other knee in. Bring the feet together so the toes are lightly touching but knees stay hip-width apart.

5. Breathe in wide.

6. Breathe out and still zipping as necessary to keep your back anchored, lower the first leg you raised.

7. Breathe in, then out and lower the second leg.

Repeat six times, alternating which leg you raise and lower first.

When you are confident that you have mastered level 2, then you may raise and lower both legs, still one at a time, but on a single out-breath.

ACTION FOR TURNING THE LEG OUT

To learn how to turn the leg out of the hip joint with stability, please refer to The Oyster (page 78).

Watchpoints

As for Single Knee Folds and Double Knee Folds, level 1, plus:
- Keep your sacrum anchored and square on the mat, the tailbone down.
- Keep the back of your neck long.
- Your lower abdominals must stay hollow and scooped throughout.
- Avoid any gripping in the back muscles.

upper body basics

Moving up the body now, we need to look at good upper body movement skills.

The following exercises will help you to:

Release tension in the neck and shoulders.

Learn good head, neck and shoulder alignment.

Learn how to move the arms freely – good scapulohumeral rhythm.

Strengthen the muscles which stabilise the shoulder-blades.

Learn how to stabilise the cervical spine with the cervical nod.

floating arms

AIM

We all have a tendency to overuse the upper part of our shoulders, which tends to create unwanted tension. What we are aiming for is smooth, flowing movement as your arm rises. As you lift your arm, think of this order of movement:

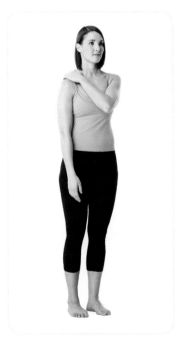

1. Just your arm moves up and out.

2. Then you will feel the shoulder-blade start to move – it coils down and around the back of the ribcage.

3. Finally the collarbone will raise up.

Starting Position

Stand tall. Place your left hand on your right shoulder – feel your collarbone. You are going to try to keep the collarbone still for the first part of the movement, your hand checking that the upper part of your shoulder remains 'quiet' for as long as possible. Very often this part will overwork, so think of it staying soft and released.

ACTION

1. Breathe in to prepare and lengthen up through the spine, letting the neck relax.

2. Breathe out, gentle zip, as you raise the arm, keeping it within your peripheral vision. As the arm reaches shoulder level, rotate it so that the palm opens to the ceiling. Try to keep the upper shoulder under your hand as still as possible. Think of the order of movement shown on the opposite page.

3. Breathe in and hold the arm lifted.

4. Breathe out as you lower the arm with control.

Repeat three times with each arm.

Watchpoints

- Do keep sight of the working arm to avoid any impingement on the shoulder joint.
- Do not fix the shoulder-blades down into the back. They will naturally glide down and around as the arm lifts, but do keep the distance between the ears and the shoulders. Do not allow the shoulder to hike up.
- Keep a sense of openness in the front and back of the upper body.
- Do not allow your body to shift to the side. Keep centred.
- Think of the hand as leading the arm and the arm as following the hand as it floats upwards.

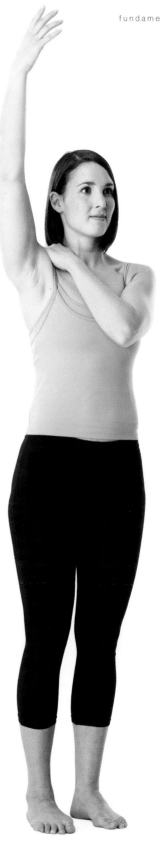

the dart preparation

In this exercise we are going to use the opening stage of the Dart (you'll find
the full version and variation on page 102) to help you to feel what we mean
by opening across the chest and also helping you to locate the muscles
which stabilise the shoulder-blades.

Starting Position

Lie on your front in a straight line. Place a flat pillow or folded towel under your forehead to allow
you to breathe. Have your arms down at your sides, palms facing up. Your legs should be
together, but with the heels relaxed apart. Open and relax your upper body. Your shoulders may be
rounded forward slightly. Notice too that your head is probably tilted forward slightly even though it
is resting on the pillow. The first action below requires you to bring the head and neck up to be in a
line with the spine. Your upper back may extend (bend backwards) a little as you open and glide
the shoulders down. Think wide and open across your collarbones and across your upper back.

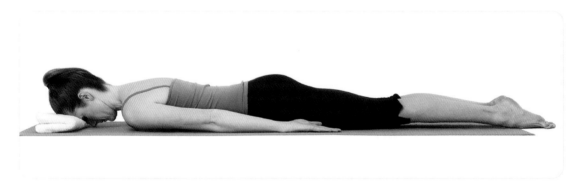

ACTION

1. Breathe in wide to the ribcage. Imagine that you have a marble on the mat by your nose.

2. Breathe out, zip gently. Lengthen through the crown of the head as you imagine gently rolling
the marble along the mat until your head is in a line with the spine. At the same time slowly open
and widen across your collarbones.

3. Breathe in.

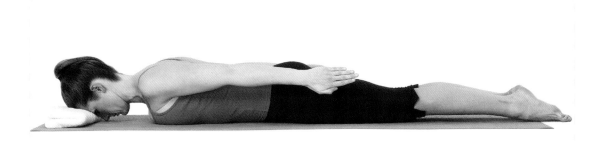

4. Breathe out and continue to lengthen through the crown of the head as you rotate the arms so that they face your body and reach through the fingertips towards your feet. The shoulder-blades will glide down your back a little as you do so. You may extend your back and lift from the floor if you wish.

5. Breathe in and hold the reach.

6. Breathe in and feel the length of the body from the tips of your toes to the top of your head.

7. Breathe out and lengthen as you release and relax.

Repeat up to eight times then come back into the Rest Position (page 107).

Watchpoints

- Keep hollowing the lower abdominals and lengthening the tailbone away. If you feel any pinching in the lower back then place a small folded towel under your abdomen, this may help lengthen your lower back.
- Do not squeeze the shoulder-blades together.
- Do not fix the shoulder-blades down into your back. They should naturally glide there. It is a small subtle movement. It helps if you think of maintaining the gap in your armpits.

ribcage closure

This exercise teaches you ribcage placement.

Starting Position

Lie in the Relaxation Position. Be aware of the head, the ribcage and the sacrum releasing into the mat. Raise your arms so that they are directly above your shoulders. Have the palms facing away from you. Just before you begin the exercise, reach both arms up to the ceiling so that the shoulder-blades come up off the mat. Then widen and place the shoulder-blades back down. Keep this sense of width throughout the exercise.

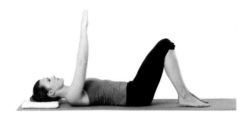

This exercise may also be done with the palms facing each other if it is more comfortable.

ACTION

1. Breathe into the sides and back of the ribcage. Feel the ribcage expanding on the mat beneath you.

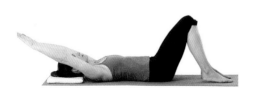

2. Breathe out, zip gently and staying zipped, raise both arms over your head towards the floor behind you. Do not allow the ribs to flare out, they should stay integrated down into your waist. Do not force the arms further than is comfortable.

3. Breathe in, return the arms to above the shoulders and feel the back of the ribcage heavy in the mat.

Repeat up to eight times.

Watchpoints

- Use your out-breath to help you keep the ribs integrated with the waist.
- Check that your spine and pelvis have remained in neutral.
- The arms are lengthened, but do not lock out the elbows.
- Move the arms from the shoulder joints. If you are very flexible, you may be able to reach the floor with the upper and lower arm touching the floor together. Do not break at the elbow or wrist. To do this without the ribs flaring is a challenge.
- Your neck should stay released.
- Maintain the distance between your ears and your shoulders.

the starfish

AIM

To combine everything you have learnt so far! This demonstrates free-flowing movement away from a strong centre. As your arm moves back, think of what you learnt in Floating Arms (page 38) and Ribcage Closure (page 42, opposite). As the leg slides away, think of what you learnt in Leg Slides (page 34).

Starting Position

Lie in the Relaxation Position with your arms down by your sides and palms facing your body or down flat.

ACTION

1. Breathe wide into your lower ribcage to prepare.

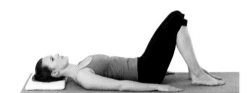

2. Breathe out, zip gently and staying zipped, raise one arm back as if to touch the floor behind. Remember you may not be able to touch the floor comfortably, so only move the arm as far as you can. At the same time, slide the opposite leg away along the floor, keeping the pelvis stable.

3. Breathe in and enjoy lengthening away from your centre.

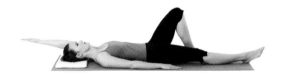

4. Breathe out and return the limbs to the Starting Position.

Repeat five times, alternating arms and legs.

Watchpoints

- Use your core muscles to control the movement.
- The ribs stay integrated with your waist as the arm reaches away.
- Think wide and open across your collarbones.
- Maintain the distance between your ears and your shoulders.

- The pelvis stays still and neutral when your leg slides out and when it slides back.
- Slide the leg in a line with the hip. Think of using the back of the thigh rather than the front of the thigh to bring the leg back.

neck rolls and the cervical nod

An important aspect of re-educating the head-neck relationship lies in the relative strength of the neck extensors (which tilt the head back) and flexors (which tilt the head forward). When sitting at a desk or steering wheel, the head is often thrust forward and tipped back, creating a muscle imbalance. By relaxing the jaw, lengthening the back of the neck and gently tucking the chin in and nodding the head forward, this balance can be restored.

AIM

This exercise will release tension from the neck, freeing the cervical spine. It also uses the deep stabilisers of the neck and lengthens the neck extensors. This is a subtle movement – you should nod your head gently.

Starting Position

Lie in the Relaxation Position. Place a flat folded towel under your head if you need one.

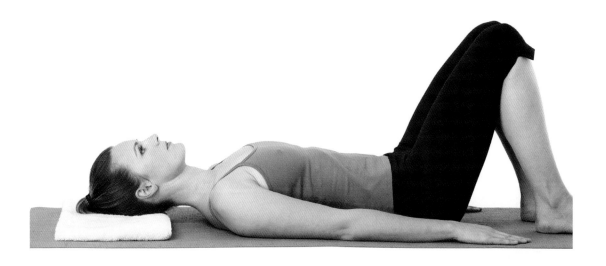

ACTION

1. Release your neck and jaw, allowing your tongue to widen at its base. Keep the neck lengthened and soften your breastbone. Allow the shoulder-blades to widen and melt into the floor.

2. Allow your head to roll slowly to one side.

3. Slowly, bring it back to the centre and over to the other side.

4. Bring the head to the centre and then gently nod your head, lengthening the back of the neck as you slide the back of your head up the mat. The head does not lift. It is a nodding action.

5. Return the head to the centre.

Repeat the rolling to the side and the nod eight times.

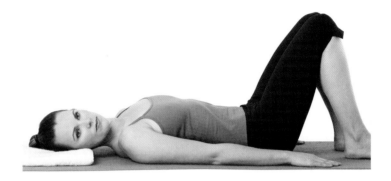

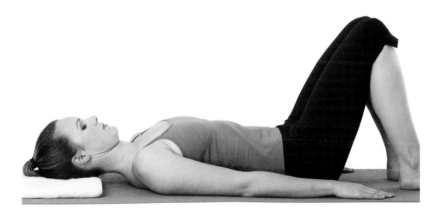

Watchpoints

- Do not force the head or neck – just let it roll naturally.
- Do not lift the head off the floor.

basic curl ups

You really need to get this basic exercise right. You may notice that there are more Watchpoints than Action points which tells you how many things can go wrong. The sad truth is that if you do this carelessly you are wasting your time. Done slowly with control, it is hard to beat.

Starting Position

Lie in the Relaxation Position. Gently release your neck by rolling the head slowly from side to side. Lightly clasp your hands behind your head to cradle and support the head – at no point should you pull on your neck. Keep your elbows open just in front of your ears throughout. Feel the weight of your head resting in your hands.

ACTION

1. Breathe in, wide to the ribcage.

2. Breathe out, zip gently and staying zipped, nod your head forward (as on page 45), soften your breastbone and curl up. Think of funnelling the ribs down towards the hips. Your lower abdominals must not pop up. Keep the pelvis level and the tailbone down on the floor lengthening away.

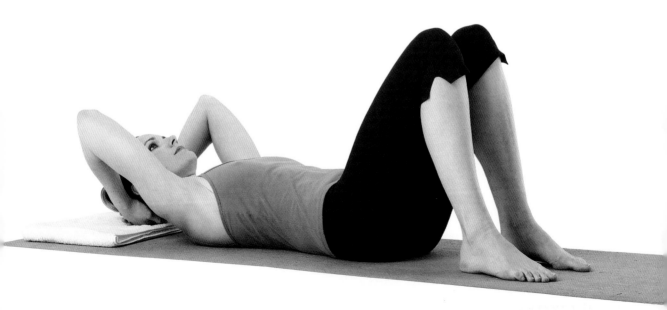

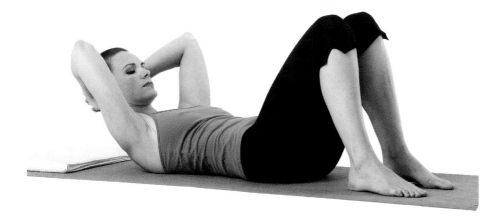

3. Breathe in and slowly curl back down again, controlling the movement.

Repeat ten times. You may add an extra breath at the top of the curl. As you do so, breathe into the back of the ribcage to keep the curl.

Watchpoints

- Stay in neutral with the pelvis tilted neither to north nor south (see page 24). The front of the body keeps its length, the tailbone stays down.
- The curl starts with your eyes, your head follows.
- Don't close your elbows as you come up – keep them open but within your peripheral vision.
- Keep the head heavy in the hands. If you feel it lighten, you may have pulled on the neck. Make sure that it is your abdominals, not your neck muscles, doing the work by funnelling the ribs down.
- Keep wide and open across the collarbones and across the shoulder-blades.
- Keep the shoulders down and away from the ears.
- Do not try to come up too far – chances are you will tip the pelvis to do so.

the x factor

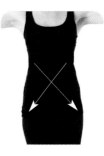

We are always on the lookout for new cues to help you move better. One of my favourites is what I have come to call the 'X Factor'. By this I mean the connection of rib to opposite hip. This forms a large 'X' across the front of your torso. It is an imaginary 'X' – you do not (with the exception of Oblique Curls) actually move your ribs towards your hips, but imagery is a powerful tool for the mind. It really does help you to stay lengthened and adds another dimension to your core, helping you to keep your trunk still as the limbs move.

the weight-loss exercises

Once you are comfortable with all the Fundamentals, you are ready to try the weight-loss exercises. It is not intended that you will work through the whole programme from start to finish, but rather that you pick-and-mix the exercises, creating your own workouts. To help you plan these, turn to the chapter on Workouts (page 108).

To help you to work at the right level of fitness for you, I have labelled exercises 'all levels', 'intermediate' and 'advanced'. I have avoided the label 'beginners' – these are simply the Fundamentals. Bear in mind that such labelling is not foolproof. We are all individuals. For example, I have always found Scissors (page 67) to be very easy, whereas Roll Backs with a Scarf (page 71) is difficult for me because of an old back injury. Some exercises have several versions, each with a different level of difficulty. You should always be familiar with, and confident with, the easiest version before you attempt the harder one.

ribcage closure with leg slide (all levels)

A feel-good exercise which will help you revise some basic skills whilst working on your co-ordination and core muscles, thus building a strong foundation for your weight-loss programme.

AIM
To co-ordinate scapular and pelvic stability.

Starting Position
Lie in the Relaxation Position. Have your arms above your shoulders, palms facing towards your feet. Keep your arms long but do not lock out the elbows. Think wide across your shoulders.

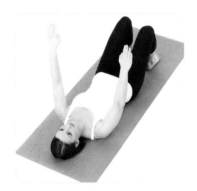

ACTION
1. Breathe in wide to the ribcage.

2. Breathe out, zip gently and staying zipped, take your arms over your head while simultaneously sliding one leg along the floor in a line with your hip. Only take the arms as far as comfortable and focus on keeping the ribcage integrated with your waist. The pelvis remains still and neutral.

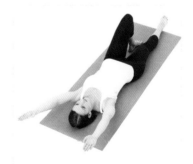

3. Breathe in. As you breathe out, bring the arms back above the shoulders whilst sliding the leg back to the Starting Position.

Repeat five times with each leg.

Watchpoints
- How far you take your arms back will depend on the flexibility and range of movement around your shoulder joint.
- The idea is to avoid the ribcage popping and flaring out. Instead, feel that the ribcage stays integrated with your waist.
- Keep your arms long but do not lock out the elbows.
- As you slide the leg back, try to use the back rather than the front of the thighs.
- Stay aware of the weight of your head, ribcage and pelvis remaining constant.

single arm fly
with knee openings (all levels)

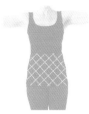

The reason this combination works so well is that as soon as you take your limbs away from your bodyline, your obliques will have to work to keep you stable.

AIM

To tone the arms, chest, shoulders and abdominals.

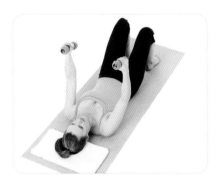

EQUIPMENT Optional hand-held weights up to 2.5kg (approx 5 lbs) each weight. Practise first without using the weights and then add the weights to maximise toning potential.

Starting Position

Lie in the Relaxation Position. Extend your arms above your shoulders, palms facing inwards and imagine that you are hugging a large tree. The arms are thus naturally curved, elbows are open.

ACTION

1. Breathe wide into the ribcage.

2. Breathe out, zip gently and staying zipped, slowly open one knee to the side while simultaneously opening the opposite arm to the side in a line with the shoulder in a 'fly' action. Your pelvis stays central and stable.

3. Breathe in and return the knee and arm to the Starting Position.

Repeat ten times to each side.

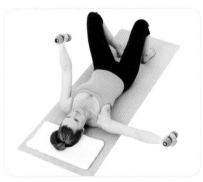

Watchpoints

- Keep the natural curve of the arm – the arm moves in one piece from the shoulder joint itself. Try not to hinge from the elbow. Take the arm directly to the side in a line with your shoulders.

- Allow your neck to release.
- Remember the X Factor (page 47), rib to opposite hip.
- Think wide across your collarbones and back.

knee folds with scarf

(all levels and intermediate level)

PART 1 (ALL LEVELS)

By adding another element to this basic exercise, you can further challenge your core.

AIM

To work the back of the arms, shoulders and deep abdominals.

EQUIPMENT A stretchy scarf or stretch band.

Starting Position

Lie in The Relaxation Position. Extend your arms to hold the scarf above your shoulders. Have your palms facing away from you, the fingers long, elbows soft. Gently pull the scarf open, connecting with the muscles which stabilise your shoulders. You should feel the back of your arms working as well.

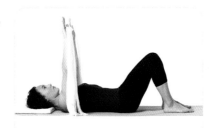

ACTION

1. Breathe in wide to the ribcage.

2. Breathe out, zip gently and staying zipped, fold one knee up keeping your pelvis still and stable. Maintain the gentle pull on the scarf. Keep your neck released and your breastbone soft. The work should be done by the muscles at the back of the arms and below the shoulder blades.

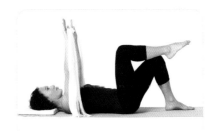

3. Breathe in and hold the position.

4. Breathe out, return the foot to the floor and release the pull on the scarf.

Repeat five times with each leg.

PART 2 (INTERMEDIATE LEVEL)

Try a Double Knee Fold. For this, you will need to turn up the zip as the second knee folds in. This will help you to keep the pelvis stable. Think of the X Factor (page 47) to help keep your trunk stable.

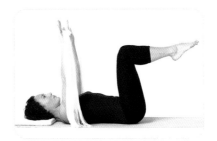

spine curls with scarf

(all levels and intermediate level)

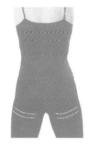

PART 1 (ALL LEVELS)
AIM

Although the primary goal of Spine Curls is to maintain the health and mobility of the spine, this popular exercise is also one of the best ways to strengthen the buttocks. In this version, you wrap a scarf around the thighs which encourages your gluteals to work even harder! The bit we are targeting is the fleshy, soft, wobbly bit of your buttocks just below your sitting bones. The outer 'saddle bag' bit of your thighs will work too as you press outwards.

EQUIPMENT A stretchy scarf or stretch band.

Starting Position

Lie in the Relaxation Position. Only use a folded towel behind your head if you are uncomfortable without one. Check that your feet are in parallel, in line with your hips and about 30 centimetres (12 inches) from your buttocks. You may prefer to move them a little closer, this is fine. Now wrap and tie the scarf around the middle of your thighs. You'll need to tie it securely, but try to maintain the legs hip-distance apart. Place your arms by your sides, palms down.

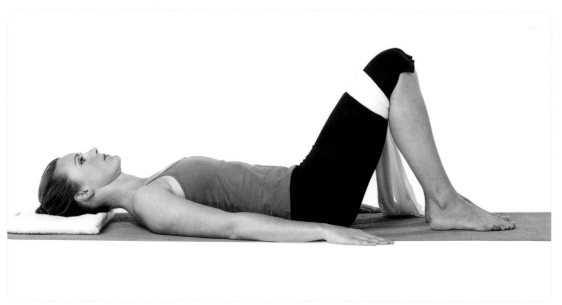

ACTION

1. Breathe in wide to the ribcage.

2. Breathe out, zip gently and staying zipped throughout, press gently outwards on the scarf and curl the tailbone off the floor just a little.

3. Breathe in, and slowly curl back down to the neutral pelvis position, lengthening out the spine.

4. Breathe out, still zipping and peel a little more of the spine off the floor – really try to open the base of the spine.

5. Breathe in and then breathe out as you roll the spine back down, bone by bone.

Repeat five more Spine Curls, bringing more of the spine off the floor each time, but keeping the shoulder-blades down on the mat. Peel up on the exhalation, inhale while you are raised and then exhale as you lengthen the spine, vertebra by vertebra, back down on the floor. Keep gentle pressure outwards on the scarf.

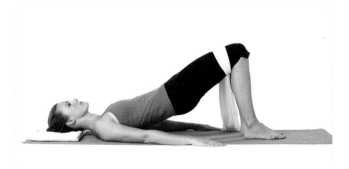

Watchpoints

- Lengthen through the knees as you curl up.
- Do not arch the back. Keep in your mind the image of a dog who has just been scolded, his tail (your tailbone) curled between his legs!
- Keep the weight even on both feet and try not to let the feet roll in or out.
- Keep lengthening the upper body too; think long from the back of the ribcage up through the crown of the head.

PART 2

(INTERMEDIATE LEVEL)

When you are very comfortable with this exercise, you may take your arms above your head, shoulder-width apart. This reduces your base of support, which will make you work harder!

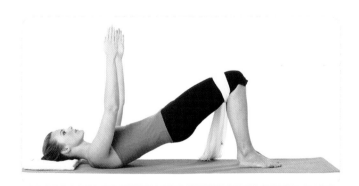

curl ups with toe dips
(all levels, intermediate and advanced level)

In this exercise, you start by learning how to knee fold in a curled up position, then progress to dipping your toes in the water! It uses the imagination as well as the abdominals.

PART 1 (ALL LEVELS)

AIM
To work the abdominals strongly.

Starting Position
Lie in the Relaxation Position. Lightly clasp your hands behind your head. Lengthen the back of the neck by gently nodding the head. Your head should feel heavy in your hands.

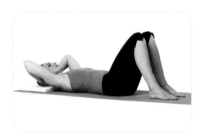

ACTION
1. Breathe in wide to the ribcage.

2. Breathe out, zip gently and staying zipped, slowly curl up sliding the ribcage down towards your hips. Pelvis remains neutral.

3. Breathe in and fold one knee up.

4. Breathe out and replace the foot on the mat.

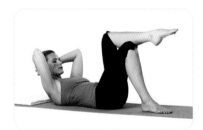

Repeat up to three times with each leg before curling back down.

Watchpoints

- Keep the pelvis in neutral throughout.
- Lower abdominals must stay hollow.
- Stay curled up. If you breathe into the back of your ribcage it will help you to keep the curl.
- Keep your head heavy in your hands, your focus stays on your lower abdomen.

PART 2 (INTERMEDIATE LEVEL)

Follow the directions 1–3 before, then:

4. Breathe out, turn up the zip, and fold the other knee up.

5. Breathe in wide to the back of the ribcage and curl up a little more if you can.

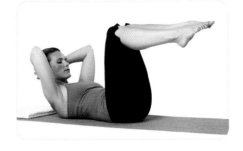

6. Breathe out, stay curled up as you slowly lower one foot back to the mat.

7. Breathe in as you lower the second foot.

Repeat up to three times with each leg before slowly lowering the legs, one at a time with control, and then curling back down.

PART 3

(INTERMEDIATE TO ADVANCED LEVELS)

Follow the directions 1–5 before, then:

6. Breathe out, strong zip, and slowly lower one foot as if to dip your toe (abdominals must stay hollow). It is a 'quick dip'.

7. Breathe in and bring the leg back to the knee fold position.

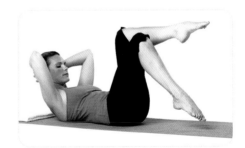

8. Repeat the dip with the other leg.

Do four toe dips with each leg before slowly lowering the upper body back down. Return the feet one at a time with control.

Watchpoints

- Move with control but do not linger as you dip the toe.
- When you are curled up, your gaze should be down on your abdomen so that you can check that it's not popping up.
- Keep the 90 degree angle at the knees as your leg lowers.
- Anchor though your centre, feel the back of the sacrum heavy. Your back must not arch.

oblique curl ups
with leg slide (all levels)

This is one of my personal favourites. I love the feeling of curling up whilst sliding and stretching the leg away. It is a common mistake when doing Oblique Curls to tip the hip up towards the shoulder rather than use the obliques to bring the shoulder towards the hip. In this version, the hip stays down as the leg slides away. Problem solved.

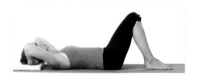

AIM

To work the obliques which define the waistline, also strengthening the deep abdominals.

Starting Position

Lie in the Relaxation Position. Lightly clasp your hands behind your head. Your elbows should be in your peripheral vision. Lengthen the back of your neck, gently nodding your head. Allow your head to be supported by your hands. It should feel heavy.

ACTION

1. Breathe wide into the ribcage.

2. Breathe out, zip gently and staying zipped, curl your left shoulder up towards your right hip, simultaneously sliding the right leg away along the floor. Think of the ribs moving diagonally around the spine towards the hip.

3. Breathe into the back of the ribcage.

4. Breathe out and slowly curl back down, sliding the leg back to the Starting Position.

5. Repeat on the other side.

Repeat five times to each side, completing ten curls in total.

Variation

Try sliding the same side leg away rather than the opposite leg.

Watchpoints

- Enjoy the opening at the front of your hip as your leg slides away.
- As you slide your leg back, focus on the muscles at the back of the thigh (hamstrings).
- Keep your collarbone wide and open.
- Do not side bend as you curl. To avoid this, keep the length on both sides of the waist.

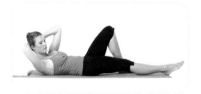

ultimate buttock toner
(intermediate/advanced level)

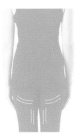

If I had to choose one powerful buttock toner, this would be it. You can actually feel your bottom tightening with every bounce. This is a challenging exercise. Please take advice if you have any injuries.

AIM

To work the gluteals and inner thighs.
To mobilise the spine and loosen the lumbar sacral area.

Starting Position

This is best done with a non-slip mat. Lie by a wall so that your knees are bent (right angles) and your feet are together on the wall. Place a small cushion between your knees. If you are very round shouldered, you may need a flat pillow or folded towel under your head, otherwise it is best not to use one. Have your arms down by your side.

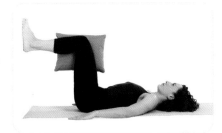

ACTION

1. Breathe in and lengthen through the spine.

2. Breathe out, zip gently and staying zipped, gently squeeze the cushion and your buttocks and slowly curl your spine, bone-by-bone, from the floor until you reach the bottom of your shoulder-blades. Hold this position.

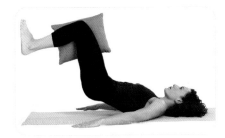

Watchpoints

- Stop at any time if you feel any discomfort.
- Keep the spine curled under.
- Keep the back of your neck long.
- Keep breathing and squeezing!

3. Breathing normally, continue to squeeze the cushion and your buttocks as you gently bounce up and down. It's a small movement. Keep squeezing and zipping. You are aiming for thirty bounces but stop when you need to.

4. On an out-breath, slowly replace the spine bone-by-bone on the floor.

Repeat three times.

the hundred
(all levels, intermediate and advanced level)

At the heart of every Pilates class, the Hundred is the most energising exercise in the programme. Designed by Joseph to 'kick start' all your body's systems, you will be working on your cardiovascular, respiratory and lymphatic systems. Here, the Hundred has been broken down so that you may learn it gradually.

PART 1   (ALL LEVELS)

Let's starts with the breathing. The goal is to breathe in for five counts, breathe out for five counts but some people find this too challenging. If this is the case, then try breathing in for a count of three and breathing out for a count of five to seven.

AIM

To learn the breathing pattern for the Hundred. To oxygenate the blood.

Starting Position

Lie in the Relaxation Position. Place your hands on your lower ribcage.

ACTION

1. Breathe in, directing your breath into your back and sides for a count of five.

2. Breathe out, zip gently, allow the ribcage to close, for a count of five.

Repeat ten times, staying zipped for both the in- and out-breaths.

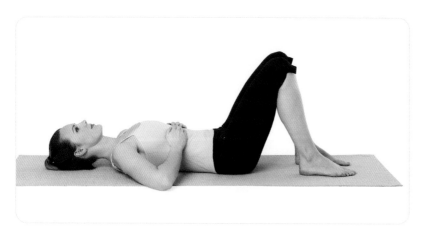

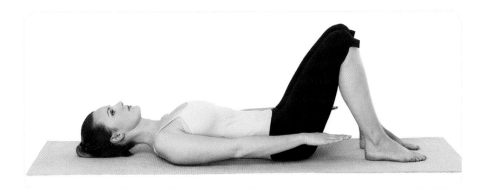

PART 2 (ALL LEVELS)

Now add the arm-pumping action which will raise your heart rate, increasing the rate that blood is pumped around the body.

AIM

To work the chest, arm and shoulder muscles.

Starting Position

Lie in the Relaxation Position with your arms placed on the mat by the side of your body. Zip gently throughout.

ACTION

1. Breathe in and pump your arms up and down just slightly off the floor for a count of five. The arms will lift approximately 15cm off the floor.

2. Breathe out and pump the arms for a count of five.

Repeat up to ten times.

Watchpoints

- Move the arm from the shoulder joint itself; your trunk stays still.
- Reach through the fingers but allow a little space under the armpits.
- Think wide across the collarbones.

- The arms are straight but not hyper-extended (locked out). Keep the wrists strong and avoid flapping the hands. The arm, wrist and hands move as one.

Watchpoints

- Remember everything you learnt in Basic Curl Ups (page 46).
- Once curled up, keep your focus down on your lower abdomen.

- Keep your pelvis in neutral, tailbone down.
- Breathe into the back of the ribcage to help you stay curled up.

Variation (INTERMEDIATE LEVEL)

This is an interim exercise to teach staying in a curled up position without the hands supporting the head.

AIM

As before but also to strengthen the abdominals.

Starting Position

Lie in the Relaxation Position. Lightly clasp your hands behind your head.

ACTION

1. Breathe in to a count of five.

2. Breathe out, zip gently and staying zipped, nod your head and slowly curl up to a count of five.

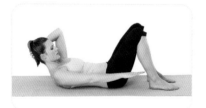

3. Breathe in and take your right hand away. Stretch it down by your side, reaching past the hip.

4. Breathe out and take the left hand down by your side.

5. Breathe in and bring the right hand back behind your head.

6. Breathe out and bring the left hand back behind your head.

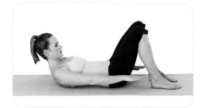

7. Breathe in and slowly curl back down.

Repeat the above sequence three times, alternating which hand you take away first.

Watchpoints

- Move the arms from the shoulder joint, keeping your body still.
- Keep your back anchored to the mat.
- Keep your focus down on your lower abdomen.
- As you breathe in, breathe into the back of the ribcage – it will help you to stay curled up.
- If it is more comfortable, open the knees a little but keep the sense of the inner thighs drawing together like magnets. The feet stay connected.

PART 3 (INTERMEDIATE LEVEL)

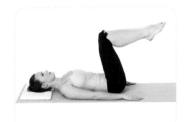

Starting Position

Lie in the Relaxation Position. On an out-breath, double knee fold one at a time with appropriate zip, toes softly pointed. The pelvis remains in neutral but your back should feel anchored to the mat. If you need to, bring the knees in a little towards you.

ACTION

1. Breathe in and lengthen through the spine.

2. Breathe out, still zipped, and nod and curl the head and shoulders off the mat.

3. Breathe in and reach your arms away from you, lifting them slightly off the mat.

4. Breathe out to a count of five, pumping the arms up and down five times. Breathe in, pumping the arms up and down five times. Pump for up to one hundred counts, inhaling for five, exhaling for five. When you are finished, slowly lower each leg, one at a time, still zipping and then curl back down.

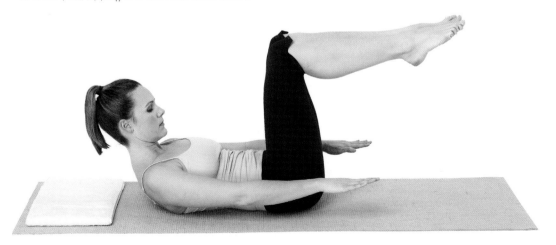

PART 4 (ADVANCED LEVEL)

In this final version, you will be straightening both legs into the air. This means that you will need excellent core control and also good hamstring length. Practise the Hip Flexor and Hamstring Stretch (page 88) to help.

AIM

To work everything!

Starting Position

As for Part 3.

ACTION

Follow all the action points before but, instead of keeping the knees bent, as you curl up, slowly extend both legs into the air at an angle of about eighty degrees from the mat (see photo below). Keep your inner thighs glued together and your legs in parallel. It is vital that your back does not arch.

Start pumping your arms as before. When you have reached 100 beats, bend the knees in and then slowly lower them one at a time, staying zipped.

Watchpoints

As before, plus:
- Your back must stay anchored firmly to the mat. If necessary, bring the legs to ninety degrees or softly bend the knees.
- Use your Variable Zip (page 27) to stay anchored.

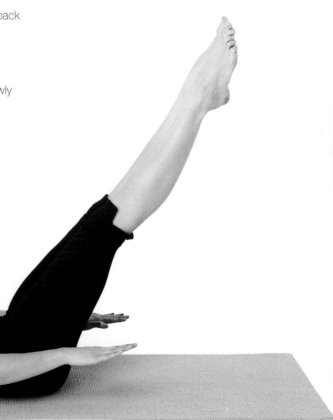

single leg stretch
(all levels and intermediate level)

A classical Pilates exercise. To master this exercise, which is learnt in three parts, you will need excellent core control and co-ordination.

AIM

To strengthen the abdominals, stretch and strengthen the legs. To learn co-ordination skills.

PART 1   (ALL LEVELS)

Familiarise yourself with the arm movement. Wrong placement of the arms closes in rather than opens out the upper body and also guides the knees inwards at the hips rather than gently guiding them towards the shoulders thus 'opening' the hips.

Starting Position

Sit tall on the edge of your mat with your knees bent in front of you. Place your left hand over the top of your right knee. Place the right hand along the right shin, as far down as possible without disturbing the openness of the upper body or causing a shift in the pelvis.

ACTION

1. Breathe in wide to the ribcage.

2. Breathe out, zip gently and staying zipped, slide your left leg away along the floor without disturbing your spine or your pelvis.

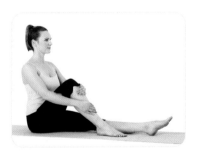

3. Breathe in and slide the left leg back, simultaneously changing the hands over to rest the right hand on top of the left knee, the left hand along the outside of the left shin.

4. Breathe out and slide the right leg away.

5. Breathe in and slide the right leg back, moving the hands across so the left hand rests on the right knee and the right hand rests on the outside of the right shin.

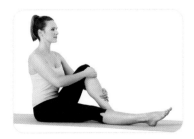

6. Breathe out and slide the right leg away and so on.

Repeat until you can move the hands into the right position, co-ordinating this with the breath and with the leg movement. Never said it was easy!

Watchpoints

- Keep your upper body open. Elbows should be soft, neck and chest muscles released.
- Maintain the gap between your ears and shoulders. You can visualise the open 'C' shape

that your arms are making. If you get the arm placement correct, the 'C' shape remains. If not, your upper body collapses inwards.
- I find thinking 'outside shin, top of knee' helps.

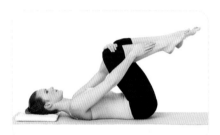

PART 2   (ALL LEVELS)

Starting Position

Lie in the Relaxation Position. Zipping appropriately, double knee fold one leg at a time, maintaining a strong centre and a neutral pelvis. Place your left hand over the top of your right knee. The hand comes round from the inside of the knee. Place the right hand along the right shin (see left). Remain lengthened on both sides of your waist. Try to keep your shins and feet parallel to the floor.

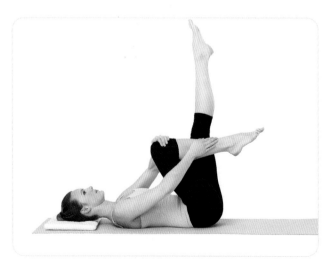

ACTION

1. Breathe in wide.

2. Breathe out, still zipping, stretch the left leg out and away from you in line with the hip, approximately eighty to ninety degrees above the mat. The leg is in parallel. Straighten the leg but do not lock it out.

3. Breathe in and bring the left leg back towards the shoulder. Swap the hand positions, reaching down the left shin with the left hand and placing the right hand over the left knee.

4. Breathe out and extend the left leg away from you in line with the hip socket, keeping the trunk still.

Repeat between ten to twenty changes, before lowering the legs one at a time, still zipping.

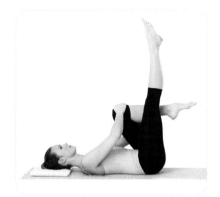

Watchpoints

- Keep the back anchored, pelvis square and the sacrum centred on the mat. If necessary, extend the leg higher into the air.
- Move the legs smoothly with control from the hip joints, keeping in line with the hip joints.
- Maintain the open 'C' shape of the arms as before.

- Softly point the feet throughout.
- Both sides of the waist should remain equally lengthened, and there should be no hip-hiking.
- Zip as necessary to control the movement and keep anchored.

PART 3 (INTERMEDIATE LEVEL)

By adding a curl up, you add extra abdominal work as well as challenging your co-ordination skills.

Starting Position As before.

ACTION

1. Breathe into the ribcage.

2. Breathe out, still zipping, nod your head gently and curl the upper body from the mat. Your hands as they were on the right leg at the start of part 2.

3. Breathe in wide to the back of the ribcage; you may find you curl up more (but keep the pelvis in neutral).

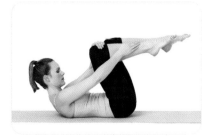

4. Breathe out and stretch the left leg out and away from you in line with the hip, approximately seventy to ninety degrees above the mat (see photo on page 66). Your leg should be in parallel, with your toes softly pointed.

5. Breathe in and bring the left leg back towards the chest. Swap the hand positions, reaching down the left shin with the left hand and placing the right hand over the left knee.

6. Breathe out and extend the left leg away from you in line with the hip socket.

Repeat between ten to twenty leg changes before curling back down and lowering the legs one at a time, zipping.

Watchpoints

As before, plus:
- Keep your gaze down on your lower abdomen so that the neck remains lengthened.
- Breathe into the back of the ribcage to help keep the curl.
- Your hands should gently guide the legs but you should not pull on them.
- You may extend the leg as low as you can but you must maintain a neutral pelvis with the tailbone down and the back anchored.

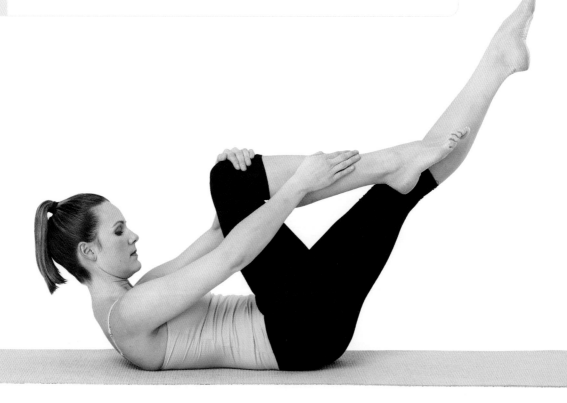

scissors (intermediate and advanced level)

A firm favourite, this exercise really strengthens the abdominals as well as the legs. It is fun too.

PART 1 (INTERMEDIATE LEVEL)

AIM

To strengthen the abdominals and improve the flexibility of hamstrings and co-ordination.

Starting Position

Lie in the Relaxation Position. On an out-breath, double knee fold one leg at a time, zipping appropriately. Take hold of the right leg behind the thigh, keeping the chest and elbows open.

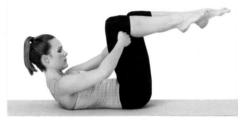

ACTION

1. Breathe in wide to the ribcage.

2. Breathe out, still zipping, and gently nod your head and curl up bringing the head and shoulders off the mat.

3. Breathe in and straighten both legs up into the air (as far as is comfortable), toes softly pointed. Now slide your right hand as far up your right leg as you can whilst still keeping your upper body open.

4. Breathe out, lengthen the left leg down towards the floor, stopping just above it.

5. Breathe in and raise the leg as straight as possible.

6. Breathe out and change arms and legs, lowering the right leg now.

Repeat up to eight times with each leg. (see Watchpoints on the next page.)

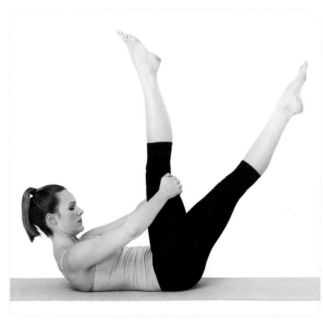

PART 2 (ADVANCED LEVEL)

When you can comfortably straighten both legs, you can increase the pace and difficulty.

Follow the Actions before but instead of a slow changing over of the hands to hold the leg, you can allow the legs to change over like scissors. As you 'catch' the leg with your hands, on the out-breath, pull it towards you with a controlled double pulse 'in in', then breathe in and stretch the leg away again. Change legs. Breathe out as you pulse the leg 'in in'. Do just five repetitions with each leg.

Watchpoints

- As you curl up, remember all the Watchpoints from Curl Ups (page 46)
- Breathe in to the back of the ribcage to help you stay curled up.
- As you lower the leg, try to use the muscles at the back of the thigh.
- Do not pull on the leg with the arms, simply guide the leg in and support it.
- The leg that stretches away must be as long as possible; keep lengthening through the toes. The leg you are holding towards you may bend a little if it is more comfortable.
- Your back must stay anchored to the mat.

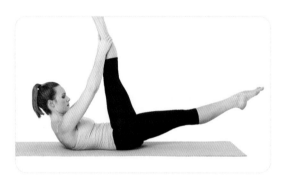

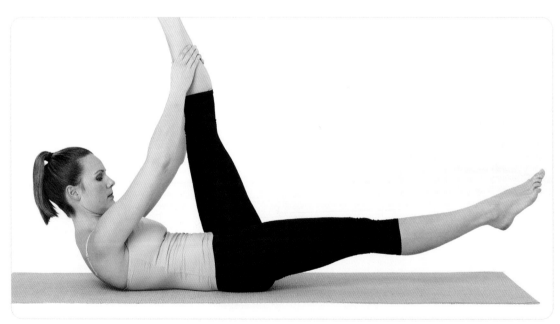

hip rolls with single arm fly (all levels)

What I like most about this exercise is that it demonstrates the need for control of movement. Done with slow control, you can feel your waist being streamlined! By adding hand weights, you can also help tone the arms and chest.

AIM

To work the waist and chest muscles.

EQUIPMENT   Optional hand-held weights, up to 2.5kg (approximately 5 lbs) for each weight. Practise first without the weights.

Starting Position

Lie in the Relaxation Position, but with the knees and feet together. Gently squeeze the inner thighs together and try to keep this gentle connection throughout. Reach the arms up so that they are above your shoulders, elbows open, palms facing as if you are hugging a large oak tree. Think wide and open across your collarbones and shoulder-blades.

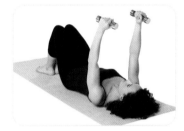

ACTION

1. Breathe in wide to prepare.

2. Breathe out, zip gently, and start to roll your knees to the right while opening your left arm to the side. Allow your head to roll to the left naturally with the arm. Your feet will roll but the right foot should stay in contact with the floor. Only rotate as far as is comfortable. Do not allow your ribs to flare.

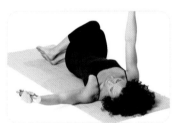

3. Breathe in wide and as you breathe out, use your abdominals to bring your legs back to the centre. At the same time, bring the arm and head back up to the start position.

Repeat eight times to each side.

Watchpoints

- Keep the inner borders of your feet, your thighs and your knees glued together.
- Maintain the natural curve of your arm as you take it to the side. The arm moves in one piece from the shoulder joint. Try not to hinge at the elbow.

star circles (all levels)

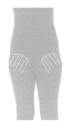

One of the things that makes this exercise so effective is the fact that you are making such small precise movements that you cannot fail to hone in on the right muscles. In this case, it's those buttock muscles.

AIM
To work the gluteal muscles and to open the hip flexors.

Starting Position
Lie on your front in a straight line, with your feet hip-width apart and legs slightly turned out. Rest your forehead on your folded arms.

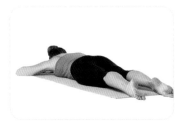

ACTION
1. Breathe in wide to prepare.

2. Breathe out, zip gently and stay zipped as you lengthen and lift one leg slightly off the mat, maintaining the turnout position. Do not disturb the pelvis.

3. Breathe in as you draw five small circles inwards, with the whole leg moving from the hip joint.

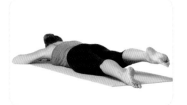

4. Breathe out and draw five small circles outwards, before lengthening and lowering the leg to the mat.

Repeat with the other leg.

Watchpoints
- Turn the whole leg out from the hip using the same wrap-around muscles you will use for the Oyster (page 78).
- Think of lengthening the thigh bone away from the hip joint.
- Keep your upper body open and relaxed.
- Try not to lock out the knee.
- Keep drawing the lower abdomen away from the mat to support your back. The tailbone lengthens away from the crown of the head. Do not allow the lower back to dip (if you need to, you may place a folded towel under the abdomen).
- For feedback, you could place the tips of your fingers under the pelvic bones; there should be no change in pressure.

roll backs with a scarf

(intermediate and advanced level)

A powerful exercise for the abdominals. Avoid if you have back problems.

AIM

To strengthen the deep abdominals and buttocks, and articulate the spine.

EQUIPMENT   A stretchy scarf or stretch band and pillow (optional).

This works better if you have a stretch band, as the band stretches to lower your back slowly. If you only have a scarf, a knitted one with a bit of give works best – you may have to allow the scarf to move through your hands a little to get the same effect.

The goal is to roll through each vertebra bone by bone. To do this you will need to engage your deep abdominals. Turn the 'zip' up as much as you need to control the movement and achieve sequential movement. As you roll back, the spine becomes an elongated 'C' shape. It is very important to maintain the length of the spine and not simply collapse back.

Starting Position

Sit tall on your sitting bones. Have your knees bent in front of you, either together or hip-width apart with a small cushion placed between the thighs. Flex your feet so that only the heels are in touch with the mat. Place the scarf or stretch band around the soles of your feet and take hold at either end with your thumbs facing upwards. Your elbows are softly bent, close to your sides.

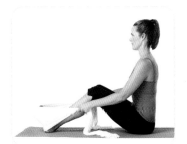

ACTION

1. Breathe in wide to the ribcage and lengthen through the crown of the head.

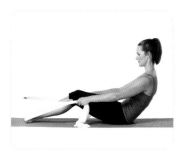

2. Breathe out, zip and staying zipped, squeeze your buttock muscles as you begin to rotate the pelvis backwards. Curl your tailbone under, sending it towards your heels. Slowly, and with control, roll the spine about half way down to the mat. Stop sooner if you feel discomfort or if you cannot control the movement.

3. Breathe into the back of the ribcage, holding the 'C' curve and scooping the abdominals back towards the spine.

4. Breathe out as you slowly roll back up, keeping the 'C' shape and leading with the crown of your head.

5. As soon as your shoulders are directly over your hips, breathe in and start to rebuild the spine from the base up, re-stacking the spine until you are sitting tall in the Starting Position.

Repeat up to eight times.

Watchpoints

- Use as much zip as you need to control the movement.
- Keep your 'C' shape lengthened.
- Keep the chest soft and open; think wide across your collarbones.
- Keep the distance between your shoulders and ears.
- Keep your gluteals working to help roll the pelvis under.
- If you are using a pillow between the knees, keep squeezing it. If not, it should feel as though your inner thighs are drawing together like magnets.
- Try not to grip the scarf too tightly, hold it firmly but avoid creating tension.

PART 2 (ADVANCED LEVEL)

When you feel confident, you can try to roll right back onto the mat. The super-advanced version would be coming back up again.

Follow directions 1–2 but this time keep rolling through the spine until you reach the mat. You will need to let the scarf out as you roll back. Your legs may straighten a little. When you try this for the first time, roll onto your side to come up again. When you have built your strength, roll down, take a breath in and, as you breathe out, nod the head and curl back up again. Keep the 'C' shape and try not to use your arms to pull you up, use your abdominals. Then follow direction 5. Repeat up to six times. Follow the Watchpoints above, making sure you keep your heels anchored to the floor.

table top (all levels)

In this exercise, you will learn how to support the body and work against gravity – it's one of the best ways to do weight-bearing strength-training without weights!

PART 1 (ALL LEVELS)

AIM

To strengthen the core muscles. To strengthen the upper body, especially the wrists and arms. Also works the gluteals.

Starting Position

Kneel on all fours with your hands directly beneath your shoulders. Your knees should be beneath your hips, your feet in line with your knees. Your gaze is directly down at the floor, so that the back of your neck remains lengthened. It should feel as though you are gently pushing the floor away with the hands.

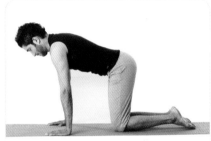

ACTION

1. Breathe in wide to the ribcage and feel the full length of the spine from the crown of your head to your tailbone.

2. Breathe out, zip gently and slide one leg away from you in a line with your hip but keeping contact with the floor. The idea is to keep your trunk still and centred.

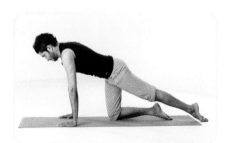

3. Breathe in and slide the leg back. Repeat five times with each leg, keeping the pelvis level and stable.

Watchpoints

- Although you will naturally have to transfer your weight onto the supporting leg, try to keep the weight as even as possible on both your hands.
- Take the weight on the whole of the hand, not just the heel of the hand.

- Think of the X Factor (see page 47).
- Maintain the gap between your ears and your shoulders.
- Your arms are straight but the elbows should remain soft.

PART 2 (ALL LEVELS)

Starting Position
As before.

ACTION

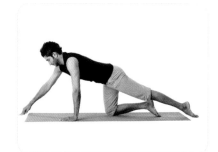

1. Breathe in wide to the ribcage and feel the full length of the spine from the crown of your head to your tailbone.

2. Breathe out, zip gently and slide one leg away, simultaneously sliding the opposite hand along the floor in a line with the shoulder. Keep contact with the floor with both hand and foot.

3. Breathe in and slide your limbs back.

Repeat up to five times with opposite arms and legs (ten times in total).

PART 3 (ALL LEVELS)

Starting Position
As before.

ACTION
Follow Action points 1–2 above, then:

3. Breathe out and lengthen and lift the arm and leg no higher than your body. The leg stays in a line with your hip, your arm with the shoulder. The pelvis must stay square to the floor.

4. Breathe in to lower your arm and leg to the floor and breathe out to slide your limbs back.

Repeat up to five times with alternate arms and legs. The most common mistake with this exercise is to lift the leg so high that you lose the neutral position of the pelvis and the spine. Move slowly with awareness and control.

Watchpoints

As before, plus:
- Keep wide and open across your collarbones.
- Do not allow your head to drop, keep your focus on the mat and ensure that the back of the neck stays long.
- Use the right amount of zip to keep the trunk still.

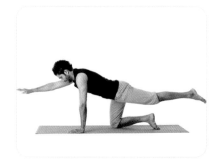

side press ups
(intermediate level)

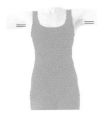

A powerful exercise which really targets those batwings! That's not to say it is just for the ladies. Men often find this quite difficult as their upper bodies are normally heavier than women's. I love the fact that you do not need any equipment, not even weights, you are simply using your body's weight against gravity. Avoid if you have neck or shoulder problems.

AIM

To work the upper arms and chest and deep stabilising muscles of the shoulders.

Starting Position

Lie on your right side with your legs slightly bent, feet in a line with your body. Place your left hand on the floor in front of you, about chest height, palm down (sometimes you have to move the hand up or down in order to get the right leverage to push up; it's slightly different for everyone as it depends on the length of your torso). Your right hand crosses your chest and rests on your shoulder.

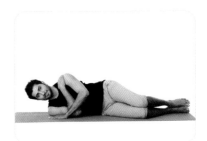

ACTION

1. Breathe in to prepare, lengthen through the body, try to connect with the muscles below the shoulder-blades which wrap the ribcage under the armpit.

2. Breathe out, zip gently and stay zipped, now press down through the left hand, straightening the arm so the upper body lifts. You will naturally twist slightly as you do this – your focus moves from forwards to down onto your hand.

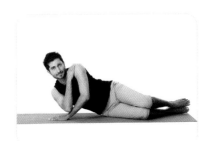

3. Breathe in and hold.

4. Breathe out, still zipping and slowly, slowly lower.

Repeat up to eight times on each side.

Watchpoints

- The slower you lower, the harder you have to work!
- Try not to overwork your neck muscles or those at the top of your shoulders. It's your arms, chest and those deep shoulder stabilising muscles which should do the work.

leg pull front preparation
(intermediate level)

This is an adaptation of the classical exercise which Joseph Pilates originally taught. It is a very powerful exercise which requires excellent upper body strength and core control. It's unrivalled for toning arms and shoulders.

Practise Table Top (page 73) before attempting this exercise.

AIM
To work the core muscles and develop upper body strength. To tone the arms.

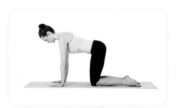

Starting Position
Kneel on all fours, your hands directly beneath your shoulders. Your knees should be beneath your hips. Your feet should be in line with your knees. Focus on lengthening from the crown of your head to your tailbone. Visualise the wrap muscles and X ribs connecting to hips. Maintain a long neck. Keep your focus down on the floor.

ACTION
1. Breathe into the ribcage.

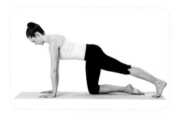

2. Breathe out, zip and staying zipped, slide the left leg directly behind you in line with the hip. When it is straight, tuck your toes underneath to take the weight onto the left foot. Immediately follow with the right leg (take an extra breath if you need to). Your back and pelvis stay still and in a long straight line. Check that your legs are in parallel and hip-width apart. The weight should now be distributed evenly between both hands and both feet.

3. Breathe in as you press both heels back towards the floor, feeling a stretch through the Achilles tendon at the back of the calf.

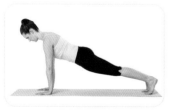

4. Breathe out as you return the heel over the toes.

5. Repeat this Achilles tendon stretch up to three times.

6. Breathe out to release the right foot and slide the leg back underneath the hip. Repeat with the left leg until you have resumed the Starting Position. Keep the pelvis still throughout. Repeat up to four times, alternating the starting leg.

Watchpoints

- Think long and strong throughout. Do not dip or sag in the middle or allow the back to arch. Keep the pelvis still.
- Keep the X Factor (page 47) – this connection will help prevent the ribs from flaring.
- Keep your elbows straight but not locked back.
- Keep your weight evenly distributed and try not to sink into your arms. Think of lengthening through the arms and lifting away from the mat.
- As with the arms, try not to lock out the knees, especially during the stretch.
- Maintain equal length on both sides of the waist.
- Zip to control, no more, no less.
- Your gaze should remain down on the mat to allow the back of your neck to stay long.

leg pull front with push ups (advanced level)

You are going to need to feel super strong for this.

Starting Position
As before.

ACTION
Follow directions 1–6, then:

7. Breathe in and slowly bend your elbows. Only dip a little way. Keep your focus on the same spot on the floor to prevent your head from dropping.

8. Breathe out and slowly straighten the elbows, without locking them or your knees. Repeat up to five dips.

9. Then breathe out to release the right foot and slide the leg back underneath the hip. Repeat with the left leg until you have resumed the Starting Position. Keep the pelvis still throughout.

Watchpoints

As above, plus:
- Turn the zip up!
- Control the movement and try not to sink into your arms. As you press up, think of lengthening through the arms and lifting away from the mat.
- Maintain equal length on both sides of the waist.

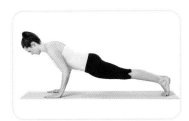

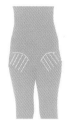

oyster (all levels)

This targets a specific part of the gluteals. It strengthens the muscles which turn the leg out from the hip and wrap around the hips. You will be using these very same muscles again and again in this workout which is why it is so important to locate them!

In this version, you use a small cushion between the knees to ensure that the right buttock muscles do the work. The movement you will be making is small and subtle but very powerful. If you cannot feel your buttocks working, stop and re-read the instructions to make sure that you are lined up properly and working correctly. You can line yourself up with a wall if this helps.

AIM
To strengthen the posterior fibres of gluteus medius.

EQUIPMENT   A small cushion.

Starting Position
Lie in a straight line on your side with your underneath arm stretched out above your head in line with your body. You may place a folded towel between your ear and arm so that your neck is in line with your spine. Place the top hand on the mat in front of you, in line with your shoulder for support. Bend your knees, placing the small cushion between them, keeping your feet in line with your bottom. You should now have shoulder over shoulder, hip over hip, knee over knee, foot over foot.

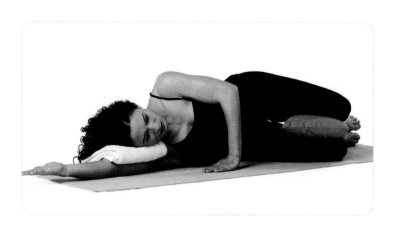

ACTION
1. Breathe in wide to the ribcage.

Watchpoints

- As you open the knee, think of lengthening through the knee while anchoring the thigh bone into the hip socket.
- The pelvis must stay absolutely still. It should not roll forward or back at all.
- Keep your waist long and equal on both sides. Normally, you should be able to slip your hand under the waist easily – you can test this to ensure that you haven't sunk into the mat.
- Your upper body should stay open and square to the front, do not roll forward.
- Do not lean into the top arm, it is there only for gentle support.
- As you open the knee keep the feet together and remember to squeeze your heels.

2. Breathe out, zip and staying zipped, open and slowly rotate your top knee, gently squeezing the heels together. Only open as far as you do not disturb the pelvis – it should stay still.

3. Breathe in and slowly lower.

Repeat up to ten times, then if you are doing a series of side-lying exercises move onto the next exercise or turn over to repeat on the other side.

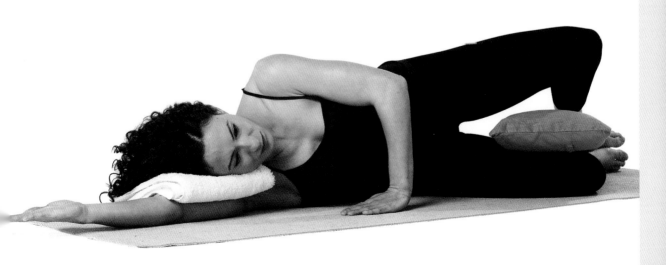

side kick front and back

(all levels and advanced level)

Great for strengthening the core, especially the waist muscles as they work to keep the trunk still as the legs move. Also works the legs and buttocks.

AIM

Mobilises the hip joints. Strengthens and stretches the muscles around the hips, especially the buttocks. Challenges the core.

PART 1 (ALL LEVELS)

Starting Position

Lie with your body in a straight line on your right side, but have your legs bent in front of you at an angle of just under ninety degrees. Your underneath arm is stretched out in a line with your body. Rest your head on the arm, using a folded towel if necessary to keep the head in a line with the spine. Your left hand may rest in front of you or on your hip.

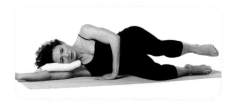

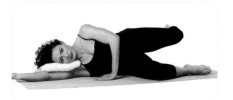

ACTION

1. Breathe in to prepare, zip gently and staying zipped, lift the top leg so that it is in a line with your hip.

2. Breathe out as you bring the leg back behind you still at hip height and without disturbing the trunk at all. Your back must not arch.

3. Breathe in, still lengthening and zipping, and bring the bent leg forward again.

4. Breathe out then take the leg back. Pelvis stays still. Repeat up to eight times, then move onto the next side-lying exercise or repeat on the other side.

Watchpoints

- Check that you are moving the leg from the hip joint only; your back must remain still.
- Remain aware of your upper body staying open and square. Maintain the distance between ears and shoulders and keep you shoulder-blades down. Ribcage connected.
- Keep the working leg in parallel and at hip height.
- Your gaze should remain in front of you.

PART 2   (ADVANCED LEVEL)

the classical front and back

Starting Position

Lie on your right side, in a straight line, shoulder over shoulder, hip over hip, and ankle over ankle, but this time have both legs forward, hinging from the hip joint, so that they are approximately forty-five degrees to the body. Keep the body still. The pelvis must remain in neutral. Place your left hand on the mat in front of your chest with the elbow bent. Rest your head on your extended right arm as shown. Zip gently now and stay zipped as you lift the left leg so that it is level with the top of the pelvis. Keeping the pelvis still, reach the leg in parallel slightly behind you so that it is extended just behind the hip joint.

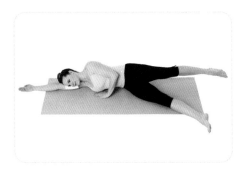

ACTION

1. Breathe in, sweep the left leg forward, hinging from the hip joint. The pelvis and spine remain stable. As you reach the end of the sweep forward, draw the leg slightly back, flex the foot, then pulse it a little further forward.

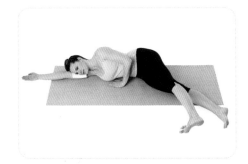

2. Breathe out, point the foot and sweep the leg back, again to extend it just behind the hip joint. Keep your back still.

Repeat six times then either move onto the next side-lying exercise or repeat on the other side.

Watchpoints

As before, plus:
- Use enough zip to keep your trunk still.
- The sweeping action of the leg should be brisk but controlled.
- Only move the leg within your own personal range of movement. Do not force it further than is comfortable.
- Keep the underneath leg active – this will help your balance.
- The X Factor will help you keep the waist long (page 47).

side-lying outer thigh lifts
(all levels)

Great for getting rid of 'saddle bag' thighs!

AIM

This exercise, together with its partner, Side-lying Inner Thigh Lifts (page 83), are hard to beat when it comes to toning the outer and inner thigh. Old favourites, they are a must in any body-shaping programme.

You will notice from the directions that a lot of measurements are given. You do not need to get out a tape measure but be aware that the most common mistake is for the working leg to be lifted way too high.

EQUIPMENT Practise these exercises without weights first, until you are totally familiar with them and they cause you no discomfort. You may then strap leg weights of up to 1kg (about 2.5lbs) onto your ankles. Start with light weights and gradually increase the load. You might also like to get a large pillow ready for Side-lying Inner Thigh Lifts.

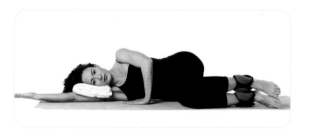

Starting Position

Lie on your right side in a straight line – this is crucial, so, to help, you can lie up against a wall to check your alignment. Don't lean on the wall! Remember, neutral. Your right arm is stretched out, your head resting against the arm, palm up or down, whichever is more comfortable. You may place a folded towel between your ear and your arm so that the head is in line with your spine. Bend both legs in front of you at an angle of just under ninety degrees. Use your left arm to support yourself in front. Throughout the exercise, keep lifting the waist off the floor and maintain the length in the trunk.

ACTION

1. Breathe in to prepare.

2. Breathe out, zip and staying zipped, lift the top leg to hip height (just a few centimetres) and take it back, straightening it so that it is in a line with your hip and your body (about 12cm off the floor). Be careful not to take it behind you.

3. Breathe in and slowly rotate the whole leg in slightly from the hip; the pelvis stays still. Flex the foot towards your face.

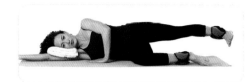

4. Breathe out as you slowly lift the leg about 15cm, then breathe in and lower it to hip height (not to the floor). Do not disturb the pelvis.

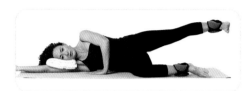

5. Raise and lower the leg ten times. Exhale as you lift the leg, inhale as you lower. Then bend the leg and rest it on the underneath leg again. Move on to the next side-lying exercise or repeat on the other side. You may also do this exercise with the working leg in parallel.

Watchpoints

- Keep zipping to protect the lower back and prevent it from arching or the waist dropping down to the floor.
- Lengthen the heel as far away as possible from the hip – think long, long leg.
- Keep the rotation inward from the hip – be careful not to turn it in just from the ankle.

- Keep lifting the waist off the floor and lengthening in the body – think long, long waist.
- Your pelvis should remain absolutely still – do not allow it to roll forward or rock around.
- Don't forget to keep the upper body open and shoulder-blades down into your back. Do not allow yourself to roll forward.

side-lying inner thigh lifts
(all levels)

Unrivalled in toning wobbly inner thighs, this exercise also works your core muscles around your waist (take your hand and feel them working as the leg lifts).

AIM

To strengthen the inner thigh muscles while also challenging your core.

EQUIPMENT A large pillow and leg weights (optional) of up to 1kg (approx 2.5lbs) for each weight.

Starting Position

Lie in a straight line on your right side; you can line yourself up with the edge of your mat. Have your underneath arm stretched out, palm up or down, in a line with your body (if comfortable) and rest your head on the arm. You may need a folded towel under your head to keep it in line with your spine. Now bring the top leg forward without disturbing the back, to rest on the large pillow. You may need a couple of pillows to keep the pelvis square. Your left hand should be in front of your chest; it is there to gently support you and help your balance. The underneath leg will be the working leg. Bring it forward slightly and turn it out from the hip joint. Softly point the toe. Take a moment to check that your spine is lengthened and still has its natural curves. The pelvis is neutral and your waist is long and lifted.

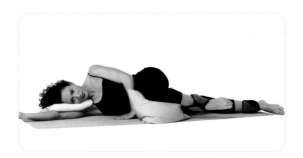

ACTION

1. Breathe in to prepare.

2. Breathe out, zip and staying zipped, lengthen and lift the underneath leg as far as you can without the pelvis or spine moving.

3. Breathe in to lower the leg to the floor.

4. Breathe out to lengthen and lift the leg.

Repeat up to ten times, rest for thirty seconds, then repeat another ten times. Turn over to repeat on the other side or start the whole side-lying series on the other side.

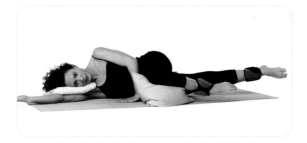

Watchpoints

- Do not collapse between lifts, keep lengthening from the crown of your head to your tailbone and then from the hip through to the toes.
- Keep your pelvis stable and still and square.
- Both sides of your waist remain lengthened and lifted. Think of the X Factor! (page 47)

- Try not to lean into the supporting arm.
- Keep your upper body open and square; do not roll forward.
- Maintain the distance between your ears and your shoulders.

torpedo (all levels and intermediate level)

Torpedo is by far the best waist-whittling exercise in the world! Part 2 requires a lot of core strength to lift both legs simultaneously from the floor so please practise Part 1 first, then when it becomes easy you can try Part 2.

PART 1 (ALL LEVELS)

AIM

To work the waistline and core.

Starting Position
Lie in a straight line on your side, your legs stretched out in parallel in a line with your body or, bring the legs forward slightly hinging from the hips as this makes the exercise easier (see photos right). Toes softly pointed. Extend your underneath arm under your head in line with your torso; the top arm bends in front of you to support you. Your other hand may be in a line with your chest or waist, your shoulder-blade down into the back, elbow open.

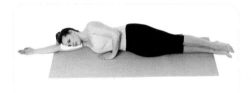
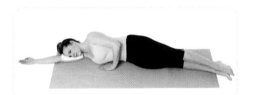

ACTION

1. Breathe in wide to the ribcage.

2. Breathe out, zip and staying zipped, lift the top leg as high as you can without tipping the pelvis.

3. Breathe in and bring the underneath leg up to meet the top leg. Make sure your legs are not behind you.

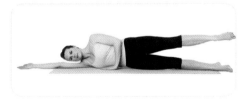

4. Breathe out and, squeezing both legs together, slowly lower the legs to the floor, resisting slightly with the underneath leg as you lower.

Repeat up to ten times then either move onto the next side-lying exercise or repeat on the other side. See Watchpoints on the next page.

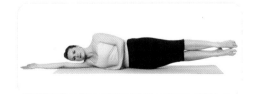

PART 2 (INTERMEDIATE LEVEL)

Starting Position
As before.

ACTION

1. Breathe in wide to the ribcage.

2. Breathe out, zip and stay zipped.

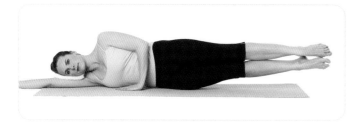

3. Breathe in and lift both legs straight off the mat as high as you can without tipping the pelvis.

4. Breathe out and lift the top leg higher, lengthening the thigh bone away from the hip. The underneath leg stays lifted.

5. Breathe in and bring the legs together but still lifted. Keep lengthening and do not allow the back to arch or the waist to drop.

6. Breathe out and lower both legs, squeezing them together and resisting slightly with the lower leg as you lower.

Repeat up to ten times, then move onto the next exercise or repeat on the other side.

Watchpoints

- Make sure that your legs are not behind you; they should be in a line with your body or hinged forward.
- Do not lift the top leg so high that you disturb the pelvis. It should remain neutral.
- Keep the waist lengthened and lifted; this is vital.
- Try not to use the supporting arm to push yourself up.
- Keep an open elbow on the supporting arm; the shoulder should stay down.
- Really enjoy the lengthening through the whole body, keeping a long waist line. Think of the X Factor (page 47).

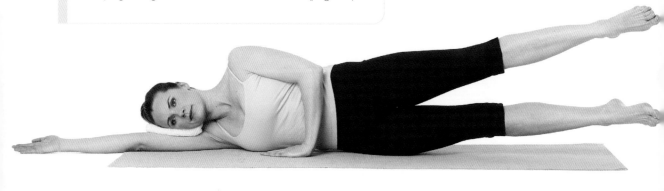

torpedo with abductor lifts (advanced level)

This exercise works to the power of three! Needless to say, it is very challenging.

AIM

To work the waistline, the core, and inner and outer thigh muscles.

Starting Position

Lie in a straight line on your side, your legs stretched out in parallel in a line with your body or brought forward slightly, hinging from the hips as this makes the exercise easier (see top two photos). Toes softly pointed. Extend your underneath arm under your head in line with your torso. The top arm bends in front of you to support you.

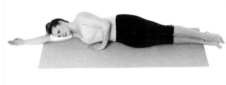

ACTION

1. Breathe in wide to the ribcage.

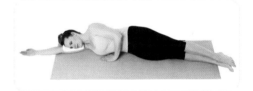

2. Breathe out, zip and stay zipped.

3. Breathe in and lift both legs straight off the mat as high as you can without tipping the pelvis.

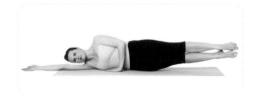

4. Breathe out for a count of five, lifting and lowering the top leg to meet the bottom leg, lengthening the thigh bone away from the hip.

5. Breathe in for a count of five, and continue to lift and lower the leg. Keep lengthening and do not allow the back to arch or the waist to drop.

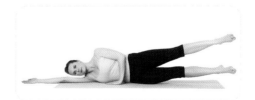

6. Breathe out, squeeze the legs together as you lengthen and lower them to the floor, resisting with the underneath leg as you lower. Repeat once more, if you can, then turn over for the other side.

Refer to Watchpoints for Torpedo Part 2.

hip flexor and hamstring stretch (all levels)

A pleasing stretch for the muscles around the front and back of the thighs.

AIM
To stretch the hip flexors and the hamstrings.

Starting Position
Lie on your mat in the Relaxation Position.

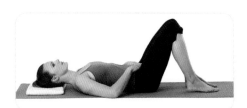

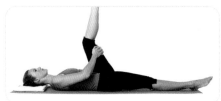

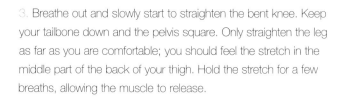

ACTION

1. Breathe in wide to the ribcage. Breathe out, zip gently, and fold one knee in towards you. Breathe in and take hold of the bent knee behind the thigh. Hug the knee towards you.

2. Breathe out and slide the other leg along the floor in a line with your hip. Breathe in and check that you are not twisted. Anchor through the back of your head, ribcage and pelvis.

3. Breathe out and slowly start to straighten the bent knee. Keep your tailbone down and the pelvis square. Only straighten the leg as far as you are comfortable; you should feel the stretch in the middle part of the back of your thigh. Hold the stretch for a few breaths, allowing the muscle to release.

4. Slowly bend the knee. On an out-breath slide the leg back along the floor and return the other leg to the floor, stabilising as you move. Repeat with the other side.

Watchpoints

- keep the knee of the leg you are stretching still as you try to straighten the leg.
- Keep your upper body open during the stretches; the elbows directed away, collarbones wide. Maintain the distance between the ears and the shoulders.

hinge back (intermediate level)

To do this exercise well, you need to bring together everything you have learned so far. Take care not to just 'lean back', you must control the hinge with all your stabilising muscles. You may like to try the exercise just once with your hands on your buttocks – you'll feel just how hard they have to work to control the movement. Avoid if you have knee problems.

AIM

To work all the stabilising muscles of the body, especially the gluteals. To work the thighs.

Starting Position

High kneel on your mat with your knees and feet hip-width apart in parallel. Extend your arms out in front of you at shoulder height, palms down. Reach through the fingers and lengthen through the crown of the head.

ACTION

1. Breathe in wide to the ribcage.

2. Breathe out, zip and staying zipped, move your body in a straight line, hinge back.

3. Breathe in and hold the position.

4. Breathe out and slowly, moving as one line, come back to upright.

Repeat up to six times.

Watchpoints

- It is crucial that you hinge back in one piece. Do not dip in the middle.
- Only hinge back as far as you can control your movement.
- Think of the inner thighs as magnets drawing together.
- Zip as needed.

high-kneeling side reach

(all levels and advanced level)

A great way to both stretch and strengthen the waist. In this version, you are also strengthening the inner thighs.

AIM
To articulate the spine in side flexion. To work and stretch the waist muscles.

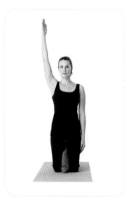

Starting Position
High-kneel with your knees in a line and a small pillow between the inner thighs. Your pelvis should be facing square to the front. Have your arms down by your side. Throughout the exercise, gently zip and squeeze the pillow.

ACTION
1. Breathe in and raise one arm out to the side and above your head. Feel the shoulder-blades widen as you raise the arm and make sure that you do not hunch the shoulders.

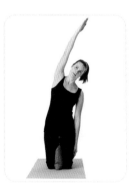

2. Breathe out, still zipping, and lengthen through the crown of the head to reach to the upper corner of the room, laterally bending the spine. Keep anchoring through both the hips and the knees (especially on the side you are reaching away from).

3. Breathe into the ribcage, focusing on the side you have stretched.

4. As you breathe out, close down that rib, keep lengthening through the head as you return to upright. Lower the arm.

Repeat four times on each side.

Watchpoints

- Ensure that you have moved in one plane only and not bent forward or back. It's as though you are sliding between two planes of glass.
- Think up and over to avoid collapsing at the waist.

- Your head moves naturally as part of the spine, so do not twist it any further. Your gaze remains forward.
- Keep your pelvis grounded and feel equal weight through both knees.
- Lengthen through both sides of the waist.

PART 2 (ADVANCED LEVEL)

adding a rotation

This version involves both the movements of side flexion and rotation. This will require great control on your behalf. Always prepare your body with a rotation exercise before attempting this. Avoid if you have back problems.

ACTION

Follow the directions 1–3 before, then:

4. Breathe out and slowly rotate your upper body, moving the bottom rib backwards, so that you end up facing the floor. Keep your arm close to your ear and your upper body twisting under you.

5. Breathe in and slowly unwind with control, bringing yourself back to upright.

Repeat three times on each side.

Watchpoints

- Keep squeezing the cushion between your knees and anchoring down through both hips.
- Keep the pelvis facing forward.
- As the bottom rib moves back, keep lifting and working through the underneath waist. You should feel a pleasant stretch on the opposite side.
- The movement back up is along a spiral.

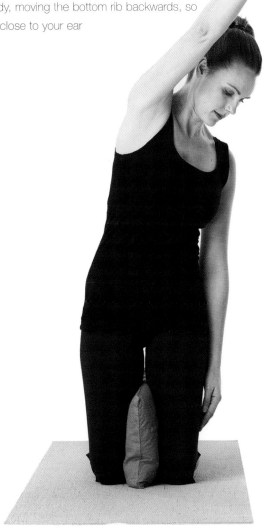

standing side reach with knee bends (all levels)

This exercise works so well because you can really get a sense of 'opposition'. By this I mean that as you are pushing the floor away through your feet, you also reach and stretch to the ceiling. It feels great. A perfect example of the opposition effect!

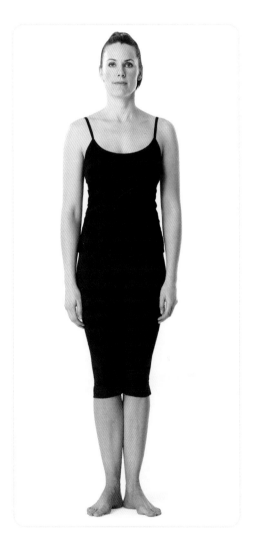

AIM

To work and stretch the waist. To work the inner thighs, wrap buttock muscles and calves.

Starting Position

Stand tall with your legs turned out from the hips. The feet are in a small 'V'. This is called Pilates Stance. Your pelvis should be facing square to the front. Have your arms down by your side. Gently zip and stay zipped.

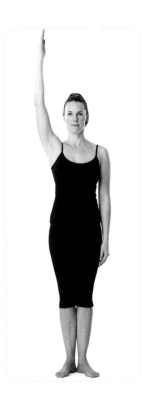

ACTION

1. Breathe in and float one arm out to the side and above your head. Feel the shoulder-blades widen as you raise the arm and make sure that you do not hunch the shoulder up as for Floating Arms (page 38).

2. Breathe out, lengthen through the crown of the head to reach to the upper corner of the room, laterally bending the spine, simultaneously bending both knees. Anchor through both hips and both feet.

3. Breathe into the ribcage, focusing on the side you have stretched.

4. As you breathe out, close down that side of the ribcage and keep lengthening through the head as you return to upright, simultaneously straightening both legs.

5. Breathe in and lower the arm.

Repeat four times on each side.

Watchpoints

- As you bend the knees, send them directly over the centre of each foot. Do not bend them too far.
- Keep the tailbone lengthening towards the floor, so that you do not stick your bottom out!
- As you straighten the knees, think of pushing the floor away evenly through both feet and drawing up through the inside of both legs.
- Think up and over as you stretch, lengthening both sides of your waist.
- Notice the direction to focus, particularly on breathing into one rib, so if you are stretching to the left, you breathe into both ribs but you focus on the right lung. Then as you breathe out, think of closing down that right rib and it will help to bring you upright.
- Keep your lifted arm in your peripheral vision.
- Remember the Watchpoints for High-Kneeling Side Reach (page 90).

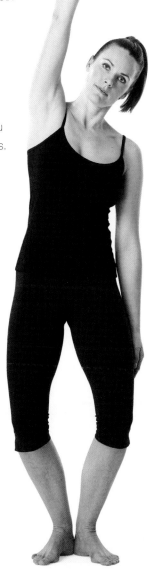

standing rotation with knee bends

(all levels and intermediate level)

Following along similar lines to the previous exercise, only this time instead of side-bending the spine, you are rotating it.

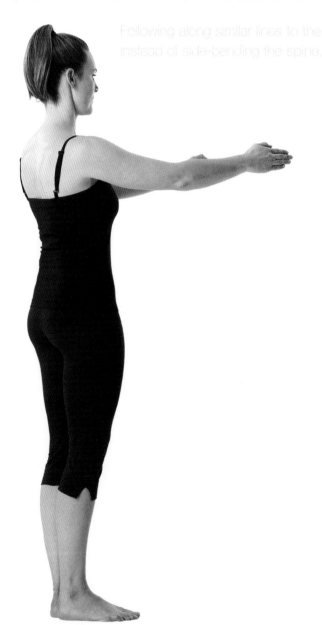

AIM

To rotate the spine with length and stability. To work the inner thighs, wrap buttock muscles and calves.

PART 1 (ALL LEVELS)

Starting Position

Stand tall with your legs turned out from the hips. The feet are in a small 'V' Pilates Stance (see page 92). Your pelvis should be facing square to the front. Have your arms out in front of you at shoulder height, palms facing in, as if hugging a large tree.

ACTION

1. Breathe in and lengthen up through the spine.

2. Breathe out, gently zip and staying zipped, rotate your trunk to the right, keeping the left arm and pelvis still, simultaneously bending both knees. Anchor through both hips and both feet.

3. Breathe in and return to centre, simultaneously straightening both legs.

Repeat four times to each side.

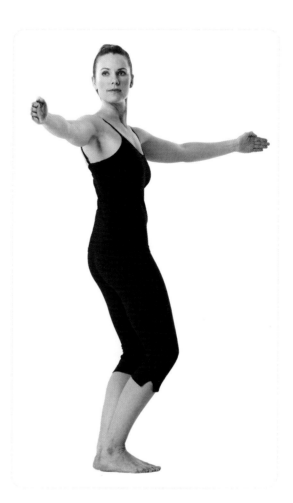

PART 2

(INTERMEDIATE LEVEL)

Turn this into an intermediate level exercise by holding light hand weights of about 0.5kg (approximately 1lb) each.

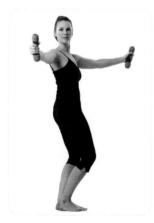

Watchpoints

- As you bend the knees, send them directly over the centre of each foot. Keep the tailbone lengthening towards the floor, so that you do not stick your bottom out.
- As you straighten the knees, think of pushing the floor away evenly through both feet and drawing up through the inside of both legs.
- Think of twisting around a central axis which is your spine. Imagine the ribcage turning around the spine.

- Your head moves naturally as part of the spine. Turn first with your eyes, head and neck down through the spine – then turn in reverse.
- Keep both sides of your waist equally long.
- Think of the arms being lifted and supported from underneath.
- Keep the arms open with their natural curve and elbows pointing outwards rather than down.

triceps and biceps (all levels)

The beauty of this exercise is that it targets both the front and back of the upper arms.

AIM

To strengthen the triceps and biceps. If using a cushion, to strengthen the inner thighs.

EQUIPMENT A weight. You can either buy a hand-held weight or use a tall can or heavy rolling pin. You can use between 1 to 3.5kg (roughly 2.5 to 8lbs) of weight. Obviously start with the lightest weight and work up. You can squeeze a small cushion between your knees if you want to work the inner thighs.

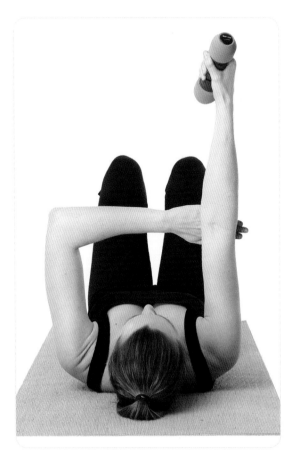

Starting Position

Lie in The Relaxation Position. Hold the weight in your right hand. The right arm is extended above your right shoulder. Palm facing inwards. Steady the upper part of the arm with your left hand. Before you begin, think wide and open across your collarbones. Breathe normally throughout.

Watchpoints

- Keep a firm grip on the weight. Keep your wrists strong and in good alignment.
- Keep your neck released and your shoulder-blades down into your back.
- If you are squeezing the cushion between your knees, be sure that you do not tilt the pelvis or grip around the hips.

ACTION

1. Slowly lower the weight down towards your right shoulder, keeping the upper part of your right arm quite still.

2. Slowly straighten the arm again, fully extend the arm but do not lock out the elbow.

3. Now turn the arm so that the palm faces away from you, with knuckles towards you.

4. Slowly lower the weight towards your left shoulder, keeping the upper arm quite still.

5. Straighten the arm again.

6. Then turn the arm back to the Starting Position, which will mean the palm is facing inwards.

Repeat the sequence up to ten times with each arm.

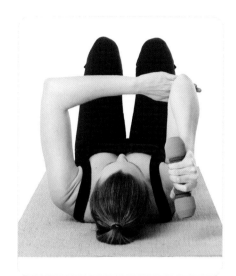

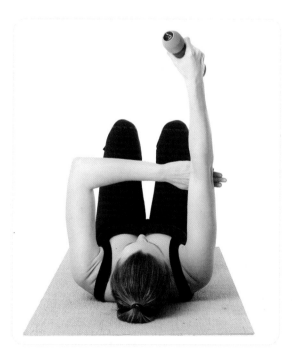

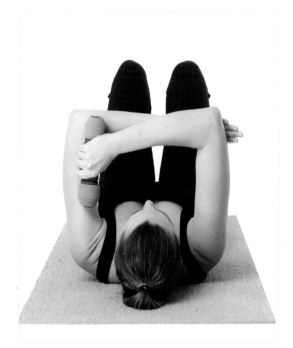

cobra preparation (all levels)

This is a key exercise in the programme. You will probably have noticed
that so far there have been a lot of exercises involving flexion (forward
bending) of the spine. This uses an extension (backward bending) of the
spine to balance your body.

AIM

To gently extend the spine and strengthen the upper back muscles.

Starting Position

Lie on your front in a straight line with your legs slightly wider than hip-width apart. Turn
both legs out from the hip joint. Place your hands palms down onto the mat so that the
thumbs are about level with your nose. Your elbows should be bent at right angles, your
collarbones wide and open.

ACTION

1. Breathe wide into the ribcage and lengthen through the spine.

2. Breathe out, zip gently and staying zipped, imagine you are trying to roll a marble away
with your nose so that your head lifts slightly off the mat and your eye focus falls just ahead
of you. Once your head is in a line with the spine, continue to curl backwards until your
chest is just hovering off the mat, thinking of the chest lengthening forward as you lift.

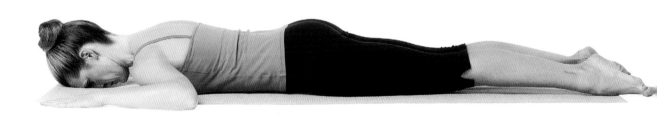

Watchpoints

- Try to use the muscles that run along the length of your spine to extend you. The shoulder-blades will naturally glide down your back as you come up but try to avoid using them to bring you up.
- The bottom of the ribcage stays down on the mat in this version.
- Your forearms should remain in contact with the floor but avoid pressing into them – that's cheating.

- Keep the distance between the ears and the shoulders.
- Keep lifting your abdominals away from the mat and lengthening the tailbone away from you. This should help to avoid any pinching in the lower back.
- If you do feel any pinching, try the exercise with a folded towel under the abdomen to support the lumbar spine.
- Avoid tipping your head back. Normally you will end up still looking at the floor, but ahead of you.

3. Breathe in and hold the position. Feel your thighs reaching away from your hips, your buttock muscles will have automatically engaged.

4. Breathe out and start to lengthen, lower and curl the spine down, maintaining the length through the spine.

Repeat up to eight times.

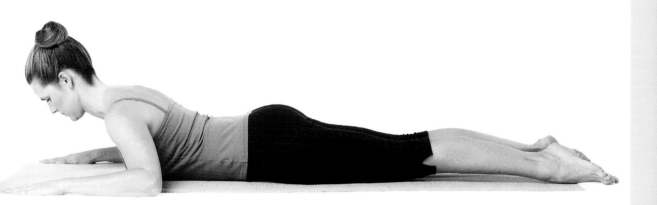

single leg kick
(all levels and intermediate level)

We are multitasking here...adding a stretch for the front of the thighs while working the back of the thighs. The kicking action in this exercise is brisk. You might want to practise a few times slowly to gain control of the movement, then speed it up but stay in control. Avoid if you have knee problems.

PART 1 (ALL LEVELS)

AIM

To stretch the front of the thighs while working the back of the thighs.

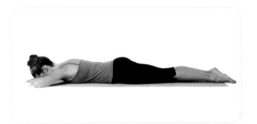

Starting Position

Lie on your front in a straight line, with your legs together, inner thighs connected and toes pointed. Place the arms on the floor in a diamond shape so that your thumbs are in the centre of your forehead. Rest your head on your hands.

ACTION

1. Breathe in wide to the ribcage.

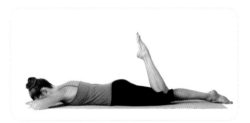

2. Breathe out, zip gently and staying zipped, briskly kick your left heel to the centre of your buttocks, keeping the toes softly pointed. Without lowering the foot, do two quick pulses with the foot – the emphasis is on the 'inward' part of the pulse: 'in, in'. Keep the non-working leg still.

3. As you breathe out, slowly straighten the leg to return to the floor as you do so, and then kick the other leg in, so that the legs pass each other as they change. Try to keep both knees on the mat.

Repeat up to eight times with each leg.

Watchpoints

- Make sure that you are kicking the foot into the centre of the buttock. Ask someone to watch if you're unsure.
- As you stretch the leg back down, lengthen through the front of the hips, but keep both hip bones and your pubic bone in contact with the mat.
- Do not allow the pelvis to tilt forward.

PART 2 (INTERMEDIATE LEVEL)

This exercise may also be done with the upper body in a Cobra Prep position (page 98). This is the original classical version. It is a very valuable exercise, as it adds another extension exercise to the programme to counter all the flexion exercises in the main programme.

AIM

As before but with an abdominal stretch.

Starting Position

Lie on your front in a straight line with the legs together. Place the hands together just in front of your head. Elbows are open just wider than and in front of your shoulders. Gently press down through the arms and slowly, leading with the crown of the head, extend by curling your upper body off the mat. Do not allow the lower back to sink into the mat – use your deep abdominals to support it.

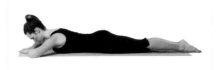

ACTION

1. Breathe in wide to the ribcage.

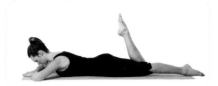

2. Breathe out, zip and staying zipped, briskly kick your right heel to the centre of your buttocks, keeping the toes softly pointed. Without lowering the foot, do two quick pulses with the foot (as before).

3. As you breathe out, slowly straighten the leg to return to the floor. As you do so, kick the other leg in, so that the legs pass each other as they change. Repeat up to eight times with each leg, then on an out-breath, slowly curl and lengthen the upper body back down.

Watchpoints

As before, plus:
- Try to use the muscles that run along the length of your spine to extend you.
- Your forearms should remain in contact with the floor but avoid pressing into them.
- Keep the distance between the ears and the shoulders.
- Keep lifting your abdominals away from the mat

and lengthening the tailbone away from you. This should help to avoid any pinching in the lower back.
- If you do feel any pinching, try the exercise with a folded towel under the abdomen to support the lumbar spine.
- Avoid tipping your head back. Normally you will end up still looking at the floor but only just ahead of you.

the dart and variations

A core exercise in any Pilates programme. It's great to have a few variations which spice it up and add extra challenge. This all serves to improve the muscle-building potential and thus the weight-loss potential. Under Action, point 4, there are a lot of directions. Familiarise yourself with each element before you attempt the exercise. It's also important to remember what you learnt in the Dart Preparation (page 40).

the dart (all levels)

AIM
To strengthen the back and tone the buttocks and inner thighs.

Starting Position
Lie on your front in a straight line. Place a flat pillow or folded towel under your forehead to allow you to breathe. Have your arms down at your sides, palms up. Your legs should be together in parallel with your toes pointing.

ACTION
1. Breathe in wide to the ribcage, imagining that you have a marble on the mat by your nose.

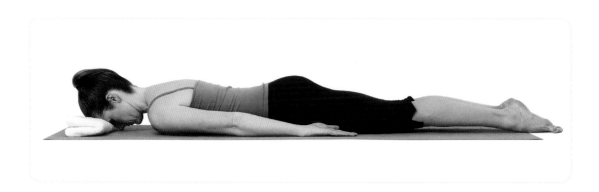

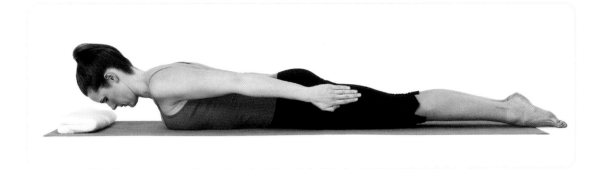

2. Breathe out, zip gently and staying zipped, lengthen through the crown of the head as you gently roll the marble along the mat until your head is in a line with the spine. Simultaneously open and widen across your collarbones slowly.

3. Breathe in.

4. Breathe out and continue to lengthen through the crown of the head as you rotate the arms so that they face your body and reach through the fingertips towards your feet. Your shoulder-blades will glide down your back a little as you do so. Simultaneously engage the buttocks and inner thighs, keep the feet on the floor and slowly start to extend the upper back. The fingers lengthen away from you down towards your feet. Think long. Keep looking straight down at the floor. Don't come up too high, just a few inches.

5. Breathe in and feel the length of the body from the tips of your toes to the top of your head

6. Breathe out and lengthen as you lower back down. Release the legs.

Repeat up to eight times then come back into the Rest Position (page 107).

Watchpoints

- Keep hollowing the lower abdominals and lengthening the tailbone away. If you feel any pinching in the lower back, then place a folded towel under your abdomen – this may help lengthen your lower back.
- Try not to use the shoulder-blades to extend your back. Use the upper back muscles instead.

- Do not tip your head back. Your gaze should remain on the mat.
- Try not to squeeze the shoulder-blades together.
- This exercise can also be done with the feet hip-width apart, either in parallel or turned out.

dart with floating arms
(intermediate and advanced level)

This variation of the Dart has the added challenge of moving the arms. This lengthens the lever and increases the hard work your upper back muscles have to do. You may either stop the arms at shoulder height or you may bring them right up above your head which would take the exercise to an advanced level.

Starting Position
As before.

ACTION
Follow action points 1–2 before.

3. Breathe in and float one arm away from your side and up to either shoulder height or above your head.

4. Breathe out and float the other arm up.

5. Breathe in and bring one arm back down.

6. Breathe out and return the other arm.

7. Breathe in and slowly lower back down, releasing the legs and buttocks.

Repeat four times, alternating which arm you raise first.

Watchpoints

As before, plus:
- As the arm floats up, try to remember everything you learnt in Floating Arms (page 38).
- You may have to turn up your zip as your arm floats up.
- Maintain a gap between your ears and shoulders.
- Keep your back extended – do not sink back down on the mat.
- Keep the head and neck in a line with your spine.

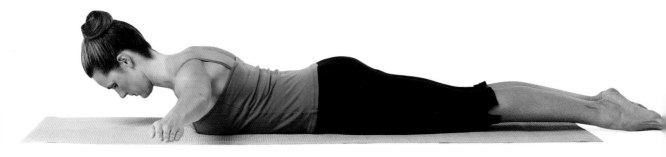

dart into side bend (intermediate level)

With this variation of the Dart, you are adding a workout for the waist as well.

AIM

To work the back muscles, waist muscles, buttocks and inner thighs.

Starting Position

As before.

ACTION

Follow Action points 1–5 from the Dart then:

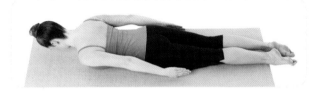

6. Breathe out, still zipping, and slide your right hand down the side of your body. Your breast bone should hover just above the mat as your upper body glides to the right.

7. Breathe in and glide back to centre.

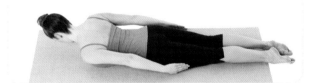

8. Breathe out and slide down the other side.

9. Breathe in and return to centre.

10. Breathe out to lengthen and lower. Release the buttocks and inner thighs and zip.

Repeat four times.

Watchpoints

- As you side-bend, try to move in one plane (do not twist or come up any higher or drop lower).
- Try not to use the shoulder-blades to extend your back, use the back muscles instead.
- Your head moves with the spine.
- Try not to squeeze the shoulder-blades together.
- Keep your feet on the floor.
- Stop if you feel at all uncomfortable in the lower back. This exercise can also be done with the feet hip-width apart and the thigh and buttock muscles relaxed.

star variation (all levels)

A good all-rounder. It targets the buttocks but also helps
to improve your posture and works the upper back muscles.

AIM

To tone the buttocks and strengthen the back extensors (the muscles that extend your back).
If you are uncomfortable lying on your stomach, place a small, flat cushion under your
abdomen to support your back.

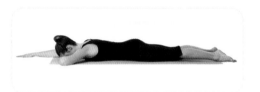

Starting Position

Lie on your front, legs turned out from the hips, just wider than
hip-width apart. Fold your left arm so you can rest your
forehead on it. Stretch the right arm out so it is just wider than
shoulder-width. Maintain a distance between the ears and the
shoulders. Keep a sense of openness in the upper body.

ACTION

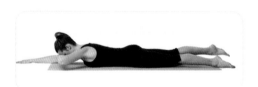

1. Breathe in to prepare and lengthen through the spine.

2. Breathe out, zip gently and, staying zipped, gently lift your
upper back. Your left arm lifts with you as does your head.
Simultaneously lengthen and lift the right leg no more than 5cm.

3. Breathe in and hold the position.

4. Breathe out and lengthen through the whole body as you lower the arm, head and leg.

Repeat five times then change arms and leg and repeat five more times.

Watchpoints

- Keep both hips on the mat.
- Think of the thigh bone really lengthening and
  reaching out of the hip joint.
- The most common mistake is to lift the leg too
  high. Think long rather than high.

- Do not push yourself up with the resting arm. Use
  your spinal muscles and mid upper back muscles
  to raise you up.

rest position (all levels)

The natural way to stretch out your back after any exercise which extends your back (bending it backwards).

Avoid the Rest Position if you have knee problems, as you may compress the joint. You may like to try a pillow under the knees.

AIM
To stretch out the back and inner thighs.

Starting Position
Come up onto all fours, bring your feet together, keep your knees apart.

ACTION
Slowly move back towards your buttocks. Do not raise your head or hands and come back to sit on your feet – not between them. Rest and relax into this position. Leave the arms extended to give you a maximum stretch. Feel the expansion of the back of your ribcage as you breathe deeply into it.

The further apart the knees are, the more of a stretch you will feel in your inner thighs.

Take up to ten deep breaths into the back of the ribcage in this position.

To come out of Rest Position
As you breathe out, zip gently and slowly unfurl. Think of dropping your tailbone down and bringing your pubic bone forward. Rebuild your spine vertebra by vertebra until you are upright, bringing your head up last. Come out of this position, slowly and with awareness.

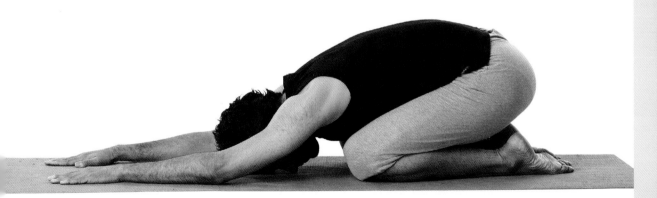

the workouts

In this chapter, we will be looking at how to put your Weight-Loss Exercises into balanced workouts. To help, I have given you three timed workouts for each ability level: All Levels, Intermediate and Advanced. The timings, 15, 30 and 60 minutes, are approximate. Follow each exercise from left to right across the page.

ALL LEVELS WORKOUTS

15 minute workout

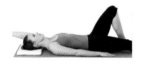

the starfish
page 43

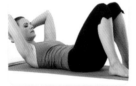

basic curl ups
page 46

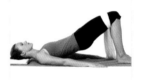

spine curls with scarf
page 52

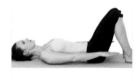

the hundred part 1 or 2
page 58

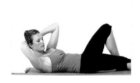

oblique curl ups
with leg slide   page 56

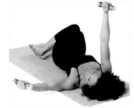

hip rolls with single
arm fly   page 69

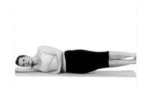

torpedo part 1
page 85

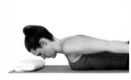

the dart
page 102

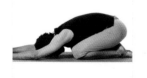

You should plan to do about 150 minutes of Pilates practice each week. Do not be tempted to do more than this, as you will be adding some cardiovascular activities (see page 138).

rest position
page 107

ALL LEVELS WORKOUTS

30 minute workout

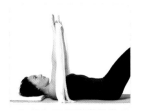

knee folds with scarf
part 1 page 51

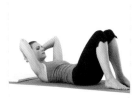

basic curl up
page 46

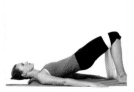

spine curls with scarf
page 52

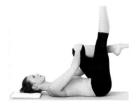

single leg stretch
part 1 or 2 page 63

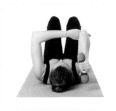

triceps and biceps
page 96

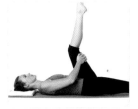

hip flexor and
hamstring stretch page 88

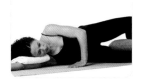

oyster
page 78

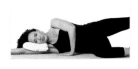

side-lying outer
thigh lifts page 82

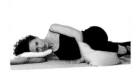

side-lying inner thigh lifts
page 83

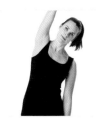

high-kneeling side reach
page 90

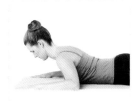

cobra preparation
page 98

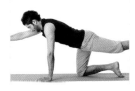

table top part 1 and 2
page 73

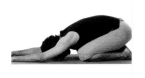

rest position
page 107

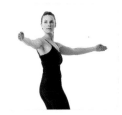

standing rotation with
knee bends page 94

ALL LEVELS WORKOUTS

60 minute workout

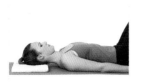

neck rolls, cervical nod
page 44

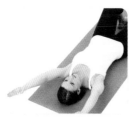

ribcage closure with leg
slide   page 49

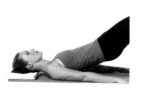

spine curls with scarf
page 52

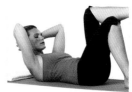

curl ups with toe dips
page 54

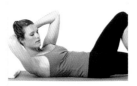

oblique curl ups
with leg slide   page 56

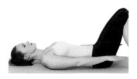

the hundred part 1 or 2
page 58

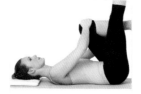

single leg stretch
part 1 or 2   page 63

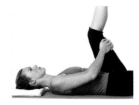

hip flexor and
hamstring stretch   page 88

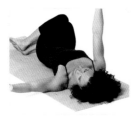

hip rolls with single
arm fly   page 69

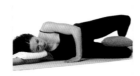

oyster
page 78

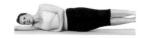

torpedo part 1
page 85

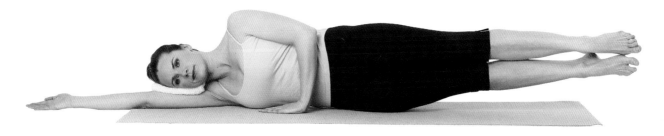

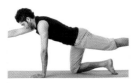

side kick front and
back part 1 page 80

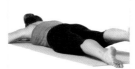

star circles
page 70

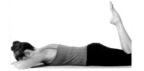

single leg kick part 1
page 100

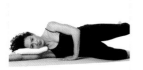

the dart
page 102

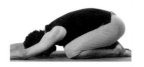

table top
page 73

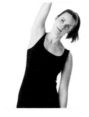

rest position
page 107

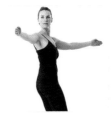

high-kneeling side reach
part 1 page 90

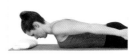

standing rotation with
knee bends part 1
page 94

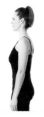

standing tall
page 19

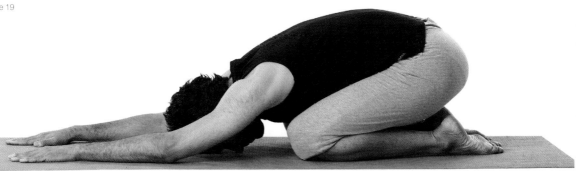

INTERMEDIATE WORKOUTS

15 minute workout

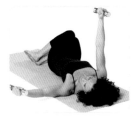
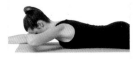
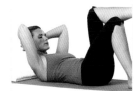
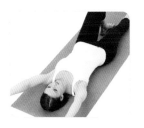
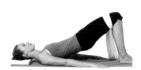
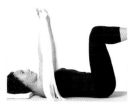
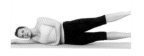
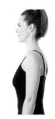
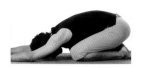
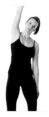

ribcage closure
with leg slide page 49

knee folds with scarf
part 2 page 51

spine curls with scarf
page 52

curl ups with toe dips
part 2 page 55

hip rolls with single
arm fly page 69

torpedo part 2
page 86

star variation
page 106

rest position
page 107

standing side reach with
knee bends page 92

standing tall
page 19

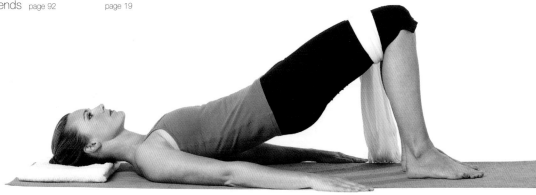

INTERMEDIATE WORKOUTS

30 minute workout

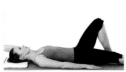

the starfish
page 43

spine curls with scarf
page 52

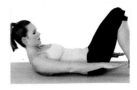

hip flexor and hamstring stretch   page 88

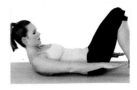

the hundred variation
page 60

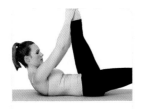

scissors part 1
page 67

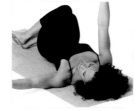

hip rolls with single arm fly   page 69

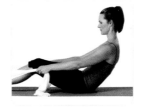

roll backs with a scarf part 1   page 71

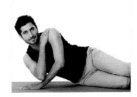

side press ups
page 75

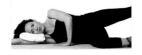

side-lying outer thigh lifts (both sides)   page 82

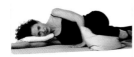

side-lying inner thigh lifts (both sides)   page 83

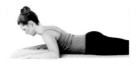

cobra preparation
page 98

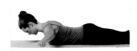

dart with floating arms
page 104

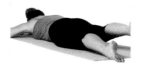

star circles
page 70

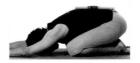

rest position
page 107

INTERMEDIATE WORKOUTS

60 minute workout

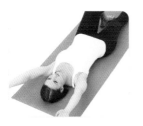

ribcage closure with
leg slides page 49

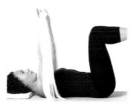

knee folds with scarf
part 2 page 51

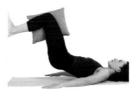

ultimate buttock toner
page 57

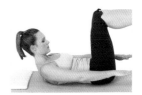

the hundred part 3
page 61

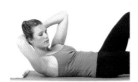

oblique curl ups with
leg slide page 56

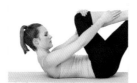

single leg stretch
part 3 page 65

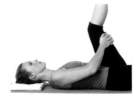

hip flexor and hamstring
stretch page 88

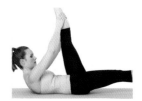

scissors part 1
page 67

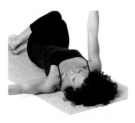

hip rolls with single
arm fly page 69

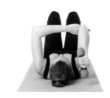

triceps and biceps
page 96

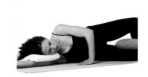

oyster
page 78

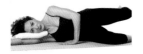

side kick front and back
part 1 (both sides)
page 80

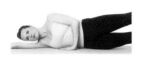

torpedo part 2
page 86

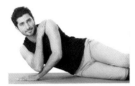

side press ups
page 75

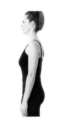

standing tall
page 19

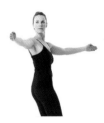

standing rotation with
knee bends   page 94

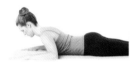

cobra preparation
page 98

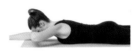

star variation page 106

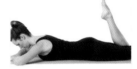

single leg kick
page 100

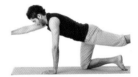

table top
page 73

rest position
page 107

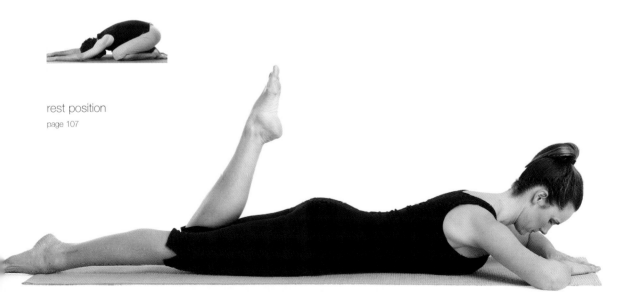

ADVANCED LEVEL WORKOUTS
15 minute workout

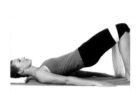

spine curls with scarf
page 52

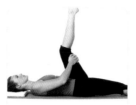

hip flexor and hamstring
stretch   page 88

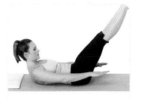

the hundred part 4
page 62

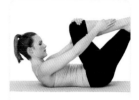

single leg stretch
part 3   page 65

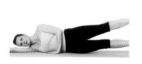

torpedo with
abductor lifts   page 87

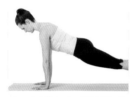

leg pull front preparation
page 76

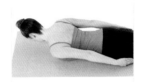

dart into side bend
page 105

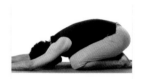

rest position
page 107

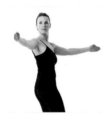

standing rotation with
knee bends   page 94

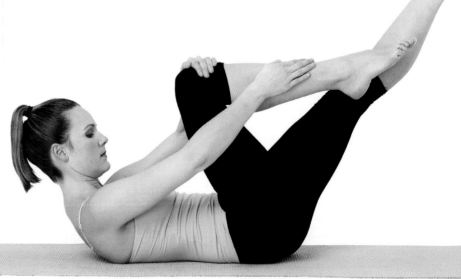

ADVANCED LEVEL WORKOUTS

30 minute workout

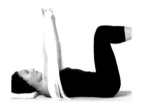

knee folds with scarf
page 51

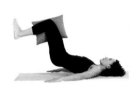

ultimate buttock toner
page 57

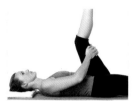

hip flexor and
hamstring stretch page 88

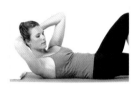

oblique curl ups
with leg slide page 56

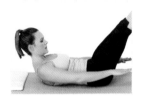

the hundred part 4
page 62

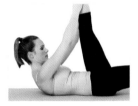

scissors part 2
page 68

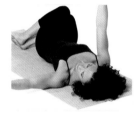

hip rolls with
single arm fly page 69

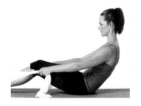

roll backs with a scarf
part 2 page 72

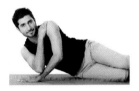

side press ups
page 75

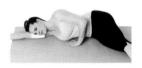

side kick front and back
part 2 page 81

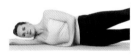

torpedo with abductor
lifts (both sides) page 87

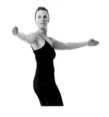

standing rotation with
knee bends page 94

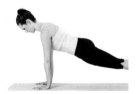

leg pull front with
push ups page 76

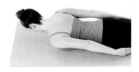

dart into side bend
page 105

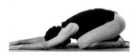

rest position
page 107

ADVANCED LEVEL WORKOUTS

60 minute workout

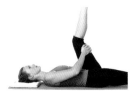

ribcage closure with
leg slide page 49

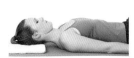

neck rolls, cervical nod
page 44

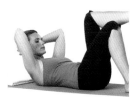

curl ups with toe dips
part 3 page 55

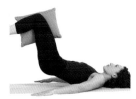

ultimate buttock toner
page 57

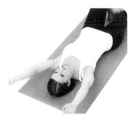

hip flexor and
hamstring stretch page 88

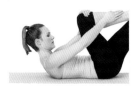

single leg stretch
part 3 page 65

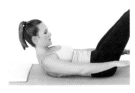

the hundred part 4
page 62

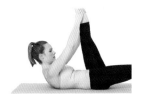

scissors part 2
page 68

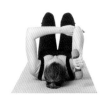

triceps and biceps
page 96

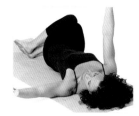

hip rolls with single
arm fly page 69

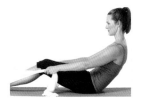

roll backs with scarf
part 2 page 72

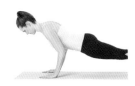

leg pull front with
push ups page 77

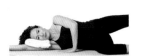

side-lying outer thigh lifts
(both sides) page 82

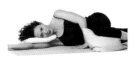

side-lying inner thigh lifts
(both sides) page 83

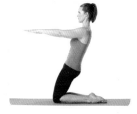

hinge back
page 89

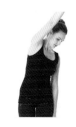

high-kneeling side reach
with rotation page 91

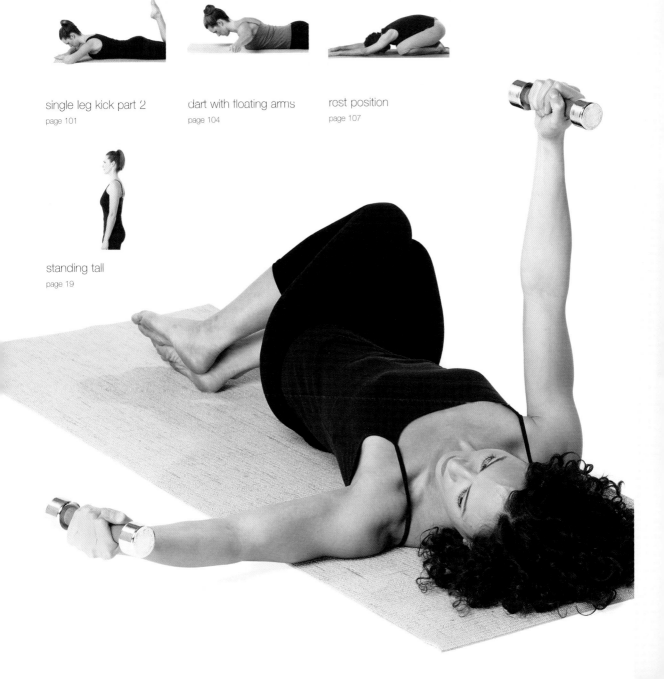

single leg kick part 2
page 101

dart with floating arms
page 104

rest position
page 107

standing tall
page 19

designing your own workouts

Over the page, you will find lists of all the exercises grouped according to levels of ability. You can draw on these lists when you design your own workouts. When creating your own workouts, you need to bear in mind the following Eight Golden Rules:

1. Plan the workout in advance and write it down. If you do not plan your workout ahead of time, you will simply end up doing the 'same old' exercises every time! Variety is key to keeping your body balanced.

2. Prepare your body. Decide how much time you have and allow a few minutes at the start to bring your awareness into your body, release tension and practise breathing. Pilates workouts do not normally need to be preceded or followed with stretches or warm-up exercises in the same way as cardiovascular exercise does. Many of our exercises make perfect opening exercises, reminding the body of how it should be moving and helping to focus the mind.

some good preparation exercises would be:

Any exercise from the Fundamentals
Spine Curls with Scarf (52)
Ribcage Closure with Leg Slide (49)
Starfish (43)
Neck Rolls and the Cervical Nod (44)
Knee Folds with Scarf (51)
Walking on the Spot (135)

3. Include all spinal movements. Even if you only have 15 minutes, you should include exercises which take the spine through all its planes of movement. By that I mean: Flexion, rotation, extension, side flexion (see box below). The extension exercises should be followed by the Rest Position (page 107).

flexion exercises:

Basic Curl Ups (46)
Curl Ups with Toe Dips (54)
Oblique Curl Ups with Leg Slides (56)
The Hundred (58)
Single Leg Stretch (63)
Scissors (67)
Spine Curls with Scarf (52)
Ultimate Buttock Toner (57)
Roll Backs with a Scarf (71)

rotation exercises:

Hip Rolls with Single Arm Fly (69)
Standing Rotation with Knee Bends (94)
High-Kneeling Side Reach with Rotation (90)

extension exercises:

Cobra Preparation (98)
Star Variation (106)
Dart (102)
Dart with Floating Arms (104)
Dart into Side Bend (105)
Single Leg Kick Part 2 (101)

side flexion exercises:

High-Kneeling Side Reach (90)
High-Kneeling Side Reach with Rotation (combined movement – 90)
Standing Side Reach with Knee Bends (92)
Dart into Side Bend (105)

upper body exercises include:

Side Press Ups (75)

Table Top (73)

Leg Pull Front Preparation (76)

Leg Pull Front with Push Ups (77)

Triceps and Biceps (96)

Hip Rolls with Single Arm Fly (69)

Single Arm Fly with Knee Opening (50)

lower body exercises include:

Star Circles (70)

Oyster (78)

Side Kick Front and Back (80)

Side-Lying Outer Thigh Lifts (82)

Side-Lying Inner Thigh Lifts (83)

Torpedo Part 1, Part 2 and Abductor Lifts (85–87)

Standing Rotation with Knee Bends (94)

Hip Flexor and Hamstring Stretch (88)

Single Leg Kick (100)

4. Balance the upper and lower body (see above). Most Pilates exercises involve the whole body. However, some are clearly targeting specific body parts. You need to ensure that you keep a balance between upper and lower body.

5. Group the Starting Positions. This is to avoid getting up and down too much. Plan your order of exercises so that you group those with the same starting position together.

6. Balance strength and flexibility. Exercises such as Torpedo, Front Leg Pull and Triceps Biceps are clearly 'strength' exercises. Balance these with exercises which 'open' and stretch you out. For oxample, Hip and Hamstring Stretch, Leg Slides, Knee Openings, Side Kick Front and Back, Single Leg Kick, Side Reaches and Rest Position.

7. Close the workout properly. Whichever exercise you choose to finish your workout, it should allow you to 'centre' yourself. Take a few moments to breathe. My favourite wind-down exercises include Starfish, Rest Position, Relaxation Position or Standing Tall.

8. Think about next time! If you can take just a moment to think about what you have done in this workout, it will help you to plan for your next workout. Listen to your body. It is very easy to repeat exercises that you find easy. Chances are that the ones you need to work on are those movements you find hard!

all levels exercise list

These are deliberately not called 'beginners' exercises because everyone, regardless of how experienced you are, can benefit from including them in their workouts.

FROM THE FUNDAMENTALS

Standing Tall (19)
Breathing with Scarf (21)
The Relaxation Position (23)
The Compass (24)
Breathing in Relaxation Position (25)
The Wind Zip (27)
The Pelvic Elevator (29)
Pelvic Stability Exercises: Leg Slides, Knee Openings, Single Knee Folds (34–35)
Scapular Stability Exercises: Floating Arms, Dart Prep, Ribcage Closure (38, 40, 49)
The Starfish (43)
Neck Rolls and the Cervical Nod (44)
Basic Curl Ups (46)

ALL EXERCISES FROM PILATES ON THE GO

Twister (131)
Dumb Waiter with Neck Turn (132)
Stair Worker (133)
Standing Quadriceps Stretch (134)
Walking on the Spot (135)
The Leg Worker (136)
Shoulder Stretch (137)
Ankle Circles (137)
Nose Spirals (137)

FROM THE WEIGHT LOSS EXERCISES

Ribcage Closure with Leg Slide (49)
Single Fly with Knee Openings (50)
Knee Folds with Scarf Part 1 (51)
Spine Curls with Scarf (52)
Curl Ups with Toe Dips Part 1 (54)
Oblique Curl Ups with Leg Slide (56)
The Hundred Part 1 (Breathing) and Part 2 (58, 59)
Single Leg Stretch Part 1 and Part 2 (63–64)
Hip Rolls with Single Arm Fly (69)
Star Circles (70)
Table Top (73)
Oyster (78)
Side Kick Front and Back Part 1 (80)
Side-Lying Outer Thigh Lifts (82)
Side-Lying Inner Thigh Lifts (83)
Torpedo Part 1 (85)
High-Kneeling Side Reach (90)
Standing Side Reach with Knee Bends (92)
Standing Rotation with Knee Bends (94)
Triceps and Biceps (96)
Hip Flexor and Hamstring Stretch (88)
Cobra Preparation (98)
Single Leg Kick Part 1 (100)
The Dart (102)
Star Variation (106)
Rest Position (107)

intermediate exercise list

Now you can draw from the All Levels list plus the following:

FROM THE FUNDAMENTALS

Double Knee Folds (36)

FROM THE WEIGHT-LOSS EXERCISES

Knee Folds with Scarf Part 2 (51)

Spine Curls with Scarf Part 2 (53)

Curl Ups with Toe Dips Part 2 (55)

Ultimate Buttock Toner (57)

The Hundred Variation and Part 3 (60–61)

Single Leg Stretch Part 3 (65)

Scissors (67)

Roll Backs with a Scarf Part 1 (71)

Side Press Ups (75)

Leg Pull Front Preparation (76)

Side Kick Front and Back Part 1 (80)

Torpedo Part 2 (86)

Hinge Back Part 1 (89)

Standing Rotation with Knee Bends Part 2 (with weights – 95)

Single Leg Kick Part 2 (101)

Dart with Floating Arms (to shoulder height only – 104)

Dart into Side Bend (105)

advanced exercise list

Now you may draw from the All Levels and Intermediate lists and the following:

Curl Ups with Toe Dips Part 3 (66)

The Hundred Part 4 (62)

Scissors Part 2 (68)

Roll Backs with a Scarf Part 2 (72)

Leg Pull Front with Push Ups (77)

Side Kick Front and Back Part 2, The Classical Version (81)

Torpedo with Abductor Lifts (87)

High-Kneeling Side Reach, Part 2 with Rotation (91)

Dart with Floating Arms (above shoulder height – 104)

sculpting workouts

In this chapter, I have given you five workouts that have been created with specific problem areas in mind. We all have parts of our body which need a little extra help. Although the workouts are balanced, you should only do them at most twice a week as part of your two and a half hours of Pilates practice. They are about 20 minutes in length. Your other workouts should be normal Weight-Loss Workouts as described in the previous chapter. If an exercise has different levels of difficulty, choose whichever level is appropriate for you.

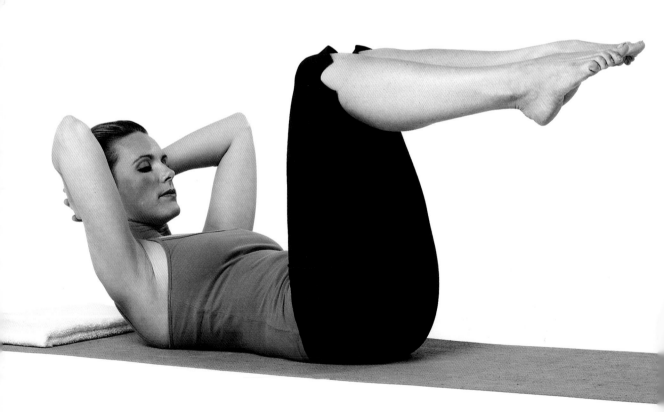

abdominals

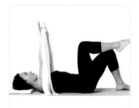

knee folds with scarf

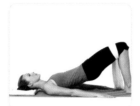

spine curls with scarf

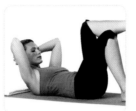

curl ups with toe dips

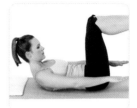

the hundred

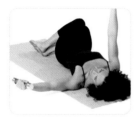

hip rolls with
single arm fly

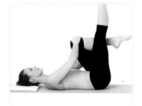

single leg stretch

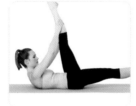

scissors

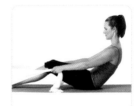

roll backs with scarf

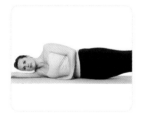

torpedo

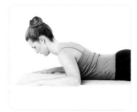

cobra preparation

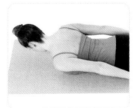

dart into side bend

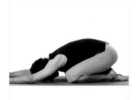

rest position

love handles

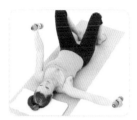

single fly with
knee openings page 50

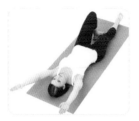

ribcage closure with
leg slide page 49

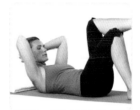

curl ups with toe dips
page 54

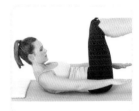

the hundred
page 58

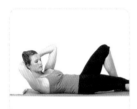

oblique curl-ups
with leg slide page 56

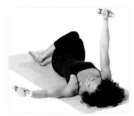

hip rolls with
single arm fly page 69

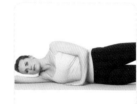

torpedo with
abductor lifts page 87

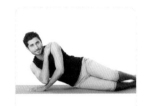

side press ups
page 75

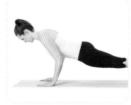

leg pull front
page 76

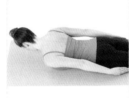

dart into side bend
page 105

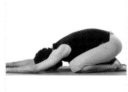

rest position
page 107

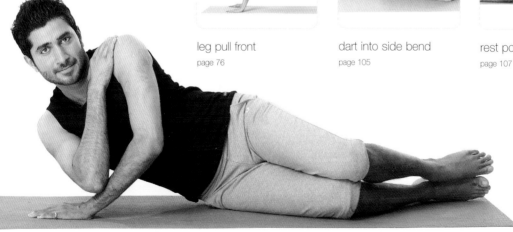

waist

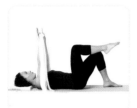

knee folds with scarf

page 51

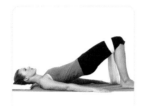

spine curls with scarf

page 52

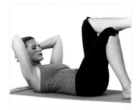

curl ups with toe dips

page 54

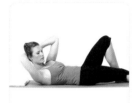

oblique curl ups
with leg slide   page 56

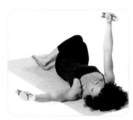

hip rolls with
single arm fly   page 69

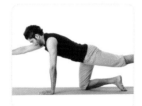

table top

page 73

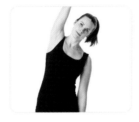

high-kneeling
side reach   page 90

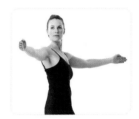

standing rotation with
knee bends   page 94

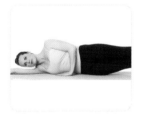

torpedo part 1 or part 2

page 85

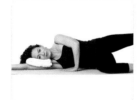

side-lying outer thigh lifts

page 82

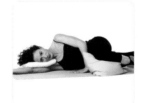

side-lying inner thigh lifts

page 83

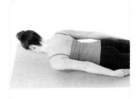

dart into side bend

page 105

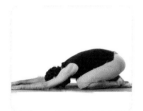

rest position

page 107

buttocks & thighs

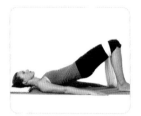

spine curls with scarf

page 52

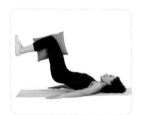

ultimate buttock toner

page 57

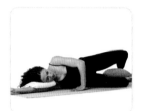

oyster

page 78

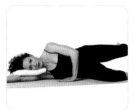

side kick front
and back   page 80

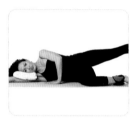

side-lying outer
thigh lifts   page 82

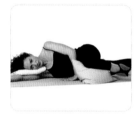

side-lying inner
thigh lifts   page 83

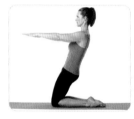

hinge back

page 89

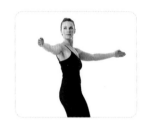

standing rotation with
knee bends   page 94

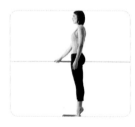

the leg worker

page 136

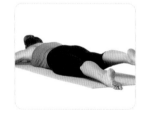

star circles

page 70

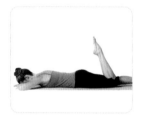

single leg kick

page 100

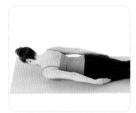

dart into side bend

page 105

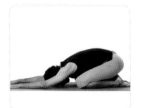

rest position

page 107

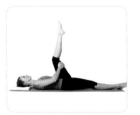

hip flexor and hamstring
stretch   page 88

upper arms

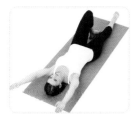

ribcage closure with leg slide page 49

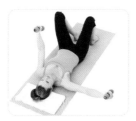

single arm fly with knee openings page 50

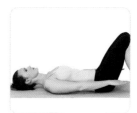

spine curls with scarf page 52

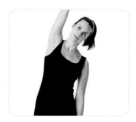

the hundred
page 58

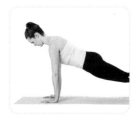

hip rolls with single arm fly page 69

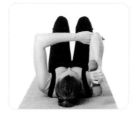

triceps and biceps
page 96

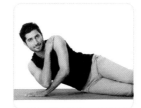

side press ups
page 75

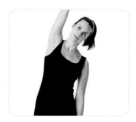

high-kneeling side reach
page 90

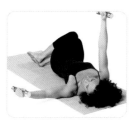

leg pull front
page 76

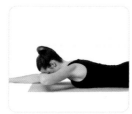

star variation
page 106

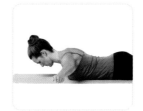

dart with floating arms
page 104

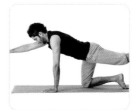

table top
page 73

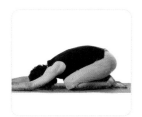

rest position
page 107

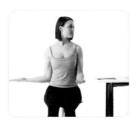

dumb waiter with neck turn page 132

pilates
on the go

Pilates is not the kind of exercise method that you can compartmentalise. It needs to become part of your everyday movements – to go with you, wherever you go. This does not mean that you need to carry your mat at all times, but it does mean that you should be mindful of your movements whenever possible.

Walk tall, stand tall and sit tall. Please do not try to stay zipped all day, but if you're stuck in a traffic jam, practise the Wind Zip (page 27) or Elevator (page 29). Be aware of tension creeping into your shoulders and neck as you sit at your desk or drive your car. Think wide and open across your collarbones. Release your neck and breathe. Then, for times when you can take a moment to yourself, here are some ideas for the office and for when you are travelling.

These exercises are suitable for all levels.

IN THE OFFICE

When you are at your desk, you might consider sitting on a physioball instead of a chair. The ball helps you to keep good posture throughout the day. Its natural instability means that your core stability muscles have to work to keep you upright and balanced. It is almost impossible to slouch as you tend to fall off! Its bounciness encourages you to stay mobile and active. Don't feel that you have to spend all day on it, even short periods of time spent on the ball are beneficial. If you cannot use a ball, try a stability cushion (page 155). This small, circular, inflated cushion can be placed on most chairs and it ensures that you are using your core muscles while you work.

Another type of chair that is worth looking at is The Swopper. Designed to accommodate dynamic movement in all three dimensions, this seat can adapt to every human movement: forward, backwards, sideways, as well as vertically (see Further Information for stockists, page 158).

AT YOUR DESK

twister

A fabulous exercise for the spine, this will also work your waist and x factor muscles (page 47). Take advice if you have a back injury.

AIM

To rotate the spine with stability. To work the obliques (you will also feel a gentle stretch between the shoulder-blades, which is blissful after spending time on the computer). For this exercise to work, you need to be sitting at your desk on a swivel chair.

Starting Position

Sit tall on your swivel chair, with your weight evenly balanced on both sitting bones. If feasible, place your feet together resting on the legs of the chair (this will depend on the type of chair. You may have to improvise and hold your feet together just off the floor. If this is the case, you will have to use your abdominals more). Hold the desk in front of you with your hands just wider than shoulder-width apart, palms down.

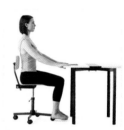

ACTION

1. Breathe into the ribcage and lengthen up through the spine.

2. Breathe out, zip gently and stay zipped. Now keeping your upper body still and facing the front, rotate your lower body with the chair. You may twist as far as you are comfortable, as long as your upper body remains squarely facing forwards.

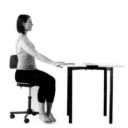

3. Breathe in, and slowly, with control, twist back to the starting position.

Repeat five times each way.

Watchpoints

- Rotate around your central axis. Imagine your spine from the tailbone to the crown of your head as a long pole which will keep its natural curves but which is fully lengthened.

- Keep the distance between your shoulders and your ears. Keeping the shoulders open and down.
- Keep the inner thighs together.

AT YOUR DESK

the dumb waiter
with neck turn

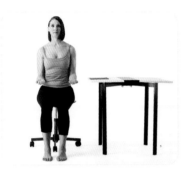

Great for stretching out the front of the chest if you have been hunched over your computer. This can also be done standing.

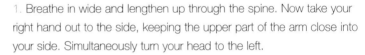

Starting Position

Sit or stand tall. Hold your arms as if you are holding a tray, palms facing upwards, your elbows close into your waist. Stay gently zipped.

ACTION

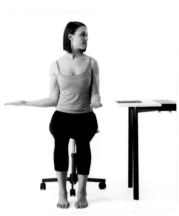

1. Breathe in wide and lengthen up through the spine. Now take your right hand out to the side, keeping the upper part of the arm close into your side. Simultaneously turn your head to the left.

2. Breathe out as you bring the arm and head back to centre.

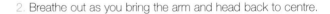

Repeat five times on each side.

Watchpoints

- Rotate the arm outwards, initiating the movement from the top of the upper arm.
- Do not pinch the shoulder-blades together.
- Keep the distance between the ears and the shoulders.
- Keep the hand, wrist and elbow in line.

- Only turn the head as far as is comfortable.
- Turn the head on a central axis. If you keep your eye line on the same level as you turn, you should avoid tipping the head back, forward or sideways.

STANDING EXERCISES IN THE OFFICE

the stair worker

A bottom step is essential for this exercise. Ensure you hold on to the stair rail or wall during the exercise. This exercise will work all your leg muscles and your wrap buttock muscles. It is quite powerful so avoid it if you have any injuries. Unless you are wearing flat, flexible shoes, you will need to slip them off.

Starting Position

Stand sideways on the bottom step so that your left leg is off the step. Hold onto the stair rail or wall firmly. Have your feet in a small 'V', legs turned out from the hip joints in Pilates Stance (as for Standing Side Reach with Knee Bends, page 92). The heels should meet on the edge of the step.

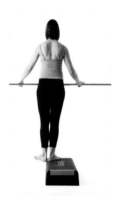

ACTION

1. Breathe in wide and lengthen through the crown of the head.

2. Breathe out, zip gently and slowly bend your right knee directly over the centre of your right foot. The left leg will lower off the step and you must work to keep your pelvis absolutely level.

3. Breathe in and hold the bend.

4. Breathe out and feel your deep wrap buttock muscles working as you slowly straighten the leg.

Repeat ten times with each leg, turning around to work the other side.

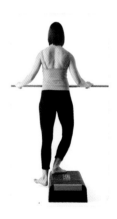

Watchpoints

- Think of the three body weights – head, ribcage, pelvis – and keep them in a line. Do not stick your bottom out.
- As you straighten the leg, push the floor away and lengthen through the crown of the head to get a sense of opposition through the body.
- As you straighten the leg, pull up through your inner thighs.
- Keep both sides of the waist equally long and think of the X Factor (page 47).

STANDING EXERCISES IN THE OFFICE

standing quadriceps stretch

As always, alignment is crucial, so do not allow the back to arch. This can be done in flat, flexible shoes, but, if you can, slip your shoes off. Please take advice if you have a knee injury.

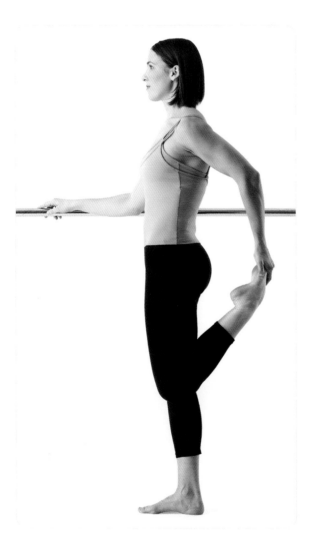

EQUIPMENT Use a scarf if you can't reach your foot with your hand.

Starting Position

Use a wall or the back of a seat to steady yourself. Stand tall.

ACTION

1. Breathe in wide and lengthen up through the spine.

2. Breathe out, zip gently, bend the left knee to clasp the ankle (or wherever you can reach comfortably). Check that you have not arched your back and that you have not shortened into one side to help you reach the foot.

3. Now gently pull the foot towards your buttock, keeping the knee in line with your other leg. Do not take it too far back. Keep lengthening from the top of your head to your tailbone. Keep your tailbone lengthening downwards.

4. Hold the stretch, breathing normally for 30 seconds or until the muscle releases.

Repeat twice on each leg.

TRAVELLING

Deep Vein Thrombosis (DVT) or 'traveller's thrombosis' has been in the media a lot in recent years. It is not that it is a new phenomenon, but it has become closely associated with flying, especially long-haul flights. There are a variety of reasons why you may be more at risk of developing a DVT during air travel, but the key factor is immobility. However, sitting still for too long (more than two hours) is in no way restricted to flying. You can in fact develop a DVT during any long-distance travel by train, car or even whilst watching a movie!

To help minimise the risk of developing a thrombosis, try to stay mobile, avoiding sitting still for more than two hours at a time.

walking on the spot

This exercise is particularly useful for getting the circulation moving.

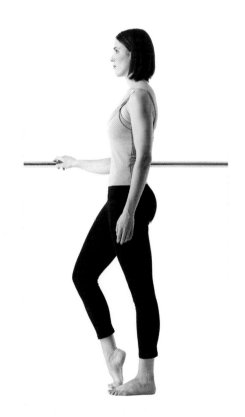

Holding on to a wall or the back of a seat, stand tall with your feet hip-width apart or together and start to walk on the spot. Come up onto the balls of both feet, then lower one heel down. Stay on the ball of the other foot, the knee then bends slightly (check it is bent directly over the centre of your foot). Change legs, transferring your weight but not wiggling your hips. Keep lengthening up, up, up, and keep the waist long.

Continue 'walking' on the spot for a couple of minutes.

You can wear your shoes for this as long as they are flat and flexible.

the leg worker

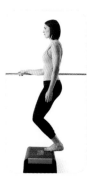

Incredibly effective at increasing circulation in the legs, this gem of an exercise also shapes them. It is best done with the use of a step but it can also be done without one. The step simply provides an extra calf stretch. Unless you are wearing flat, flexible shoes, you will need to slip your shoes off.

AIM
To work the leg muscles.

Starting Position
Stand tall with the feet hip-width apart and in parallel. If you can use a step, you will need to hold on to the stair rail – for safety, the bottom step is best. Have the balls of your feet firmly planted on the step, the arches and the heels over the edge. If you don't have a step, you won't get the stretch, but you can still work the legs.

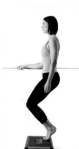

ACTION
1. Breathe normally throughout and remain gently zipped.

2. Bend both knees directly over your second toes, maintain good posture, do not tip forward or back.

3. Lift both heels so that you are now on the balls of your feet. Knees are still bent. Keep lengthening upwards, don't stick your bottom out!

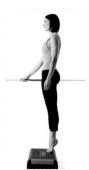

4. Slowly straighten your legs but stay on the balls of your feet.

5. Now lower your heels until, if you are on a flat surface, they reach the floor, or if you are on a step, they lower over the edge to stretch your calves.

Watchpoints

- Think of the three main body weights – head, ribcage and pelvis. Keep each balanced centrally over each other.

- Keep good leg alignment throughout. The knees should bend over the second toes. Stop and check every so often.
- Try not to allow your feet to roll in or out.

TRAVELLING

shoulder stretch

This exercise may also be done standing.

The aim is to stretch out the arms and shoulder area. Sitting or standing tall, interlace your fingers and turn your palms inside out. Reach your arms above you and allow the shoulders to come up around the ears. Then slowly draw the shoulder blades down into your back again. Do not take the arms behind your head. Repeat five times.

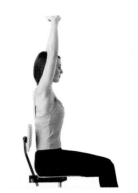

ankle circles

Sit tall. Ideally, if you have a jumper to hand, fold it up and place it under your right thigh just above the knee. It is not essential. You can also clasp your hands around the thigh instead, but keep your weight even on both sitting bones. Now circle your right foot around, keeping the rest of the leg as still as possible, rotating from the ankle joint. Make ten circles in each direction with each foot. Keep your spine in nuetral, do not use your lumbar curve.

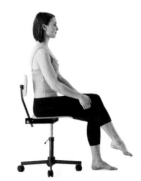

nose spirals

This is fabulous for loosening tense neck muscles.

Sit tall, shoulders open and relaxed, and with a large gap between your ears and shoulders. Imagine a small spiral just in front of your nose. Slowly and thoughtfully start to circle your nose (head follows). Start in the centre of the spiral and make the circles larger. Keep the length through the back of the neck. Keep your jaw relaxed. Reverse the spiral back inwards. Repeat five times.

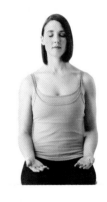

maximise your weight loss

cross-training

Although Pilates is a fabulous body-conditioning method, it is not a cardiovascular workout. To maximise the results of your weight-loss programme, you are going to need to add some cardiovascular activities.

The ideal combination would be to do two and a half hours of Pilates practice a week, combined with two and half hours of aerobic activities. This sounds like a lot, but some of your aerobic activity can be accumulative, that is, spread over the day.

Cardiovascular exercise involves moving your whole body with the use of the large muscle groups, such as the legs. It is often referred to as aerobic fitness because it uses oxygen as a source of energy to create movement and to help to strengthen the heart, lungs and circulatory system. Any activity that gets your heart working harder and raises your heart rate is a form of aerobic exercise. The cardiovascular activities you add to your programme will also help you to burn more calories.

As well as helping you to lose weight, cardiovascular activity will help to strengthen the heart, lungs and circulatory system, reduce the risk of heart disease, reduce blood pressure, improve blood cholesterol and triglyceride levels and release endorphins that will reduce stress levels.

how much and for how long?

In January 2007, The American College of Sports Medicine and The American Heart Association issued a report stating that to provide and maintain health, all healthy adults aged between 18–65 years need moderate intensity aerobic (endurance) physical activity for a minimum of 30 minutes, five days each week, or more vigorous intensity aerobic physical activity for a minimum of 20 minutes, three days a week. Combinations of moderate and vigorous exercise would also meet these requirements and it is possible for the activity to be accumulative. That is, you can do three segments a day lasting ten minutes each to reach the total of 30 minutes. This is the amount of cardio activity you need to do to maintain a healthy heart. Ideally for weight loss, you should do more than this minimum or increase the intensity.

becoming more active

One of the key factors in both heart health and weight loss is increasing your overall levels of activity. If you are looking for an improvement in overall health, even 4,000 steps a day (spread throughout the day) will help. You'll need to do 7,000 steps to improve your fitness and a total of 10,000 to lose weight. To help you calculate the number of steps you take in a day, invest in a pedometer. For your walking to count as an aerobic activity, you will have to walk at a fast enough pace to raise your heart rate.

extra toning with MBIs

One way to add extra toning is to wear a pair of MBT trainers. MBT stands for Masai Barefoot Technology. Many Pilates clients and teachers have found them to be of enormous benefit. Billed as physiological footwear, they have a number of positive effects, not only on the foot but on the whole body. By creating a natural instability underfoot, they stimulate and exercise the body's supporting muscle system. A perfect partner to your Pilates practice. They will help to activate neglected muscles, in particular the buttocks and hamstrings. Do have them properly fitted by a professional. I recommend that you wear them for just a short while to start with, and monitor the effects on your body. Visit their website for details (see page 158).

cardiovascular choices

Basically, any aerobic activity which raises your heart rate can help you to burn fat, use up calories and thus lose weight. Just find something you enjoy and which you are more likely to stick at. There are plenty to choose from, brisk walking, jogging, hiking, cycling, skiing, dancing, swimming... the list is endless. Choose an activity/class suitable to your level of fitness. Check with your doctor that it is okay for you to start a cardiovascular programme. Ensure that you are wearing the right footwear for your chosen activity. Ladies, get a good, supportive bra. Keep hydrated. Stay mindful of your posture and movements.

the training diary

Keeping a record of all the exercise that you do in a notebook will help to encourage you to exercise and also gives you valuable feedback on your progress. Record in your training diary:

Your Personal Weight Loss Plan (see page 15).
Your goals, short- medium- and long-term.
Your target heart rate for your age (see page 141).
Your workouts, both Pilates and cardiovascular.
How you felt during and after your workouts.
You can also record your weight, BMI and waist-to-hip measurements at regular intervals.

goal setting

In the opening pages of your Training Diary, you might like to record your goals again. Think about what you want to achieve over the next week, the next few months, and long-term. It may help to have specific events in mind – perhaps a date in the diary when you know you want to look your best or you need to be fit enough, say, for a charity walk or run. You can then plan and record your exercise activities, both Pilates and cardio, for each week leading up to this event.

Keep your goals simple and achievable. If you are unfit to start with, set yourself the goal of increasing the number of steps you do each day. Then, once you have achieved this, you can set another goal of making some of those steps brisk enough to raise your heart rate. In a similar way, you can set a goal of practising the fundamental Pilates exercises and then go on to start the All Levels Workouts and so on.

monitoring your progress

Review your progress weekly. If you repeatedly fail to meet your goals, perhaps you have set the bar too high? Do not give up! It takes time to change habits. Consider what may be preventing you from achieving your target. Is it time constraints? Lack of energy? If you continuously fail to meet your goals, consider contacting a Pilates teacher and/or a personal trainer for advice (see page 158). This may only be necessary for a short period of time to get you back on track.

working at the right level of intensity

We have seen that, in addition to becoming more active in everyday life, you should also include more continuous bouts of aerobic activity at the appropriate level of intensity for your level of fitness.

To find out what is the right level of intensity for you, you will need to monitor just how hard you are working and compare this with the recommended level of intensity for your age. You will know when you are working aerobically and your cells are using oxygen because you will begin to breathe harder, feel your heart beating and start to work up a sweat. It is then important to keep an eye on how hard you are exercising to make sure that you are working at the right pace for you and not overdoing or underdoing it. Exercise intensity is normally explained in terms of percentage of maximum heart rate.

how to estimate your heart rate

If you are female: subtract your age from 220.
If you are male: subtract your age from 226.

Then depending on which intensity you wish to work at, you can determine your heart rate.
Moderate intensity: 50–69 per cent maximum heart rate.

High intensity: 70–89 per cent maximum heart rate.
Very high intensity: 90 per cent maximum heart rate.

For example: a 30 year old woman will have a maximum heart rate of 190. Her target zone for a moderate intensity workout would be 50–60 per cent of her maximum heart rate or 95–114 beats per minute. Alternatively, a 20 year old man will have a maximum heart rate of 206. His moderate to high intensity training zone would be about 60–85 per cent of his maximum heart rate, which translates as 122–166 beats per minute.

age heart rate chart
A quick way of estimating what your target heart rate should be according to your age.

AGE	TARGET HEART RATE ZONE (50–75 PER CENT)	AVERAGE MAXIMUM HEART RATE (100 PER CENT)
20–30	98–146 beats per min	195 beats per min
31–40	93–138 beats per min	185 beats per min
41–50	88–131 beats per min	175 beats per min
51–60	83–123 beats per min	165 beats per min
61 plus	78–116 beats per min	155 beats per min

You'll notice that as the age goes up by ten years, the average maximum heart rate drops by 10 per cent.

The most accurate way to monitor your heart rate is with a heart monitor, otherwise you can work out your target heart rate zone by taking your pulse. Take your pulse at your neck or wrist for 10 seconds, then multiply that number by six to determine your heart rate for one minute. You will need to take your pulse around three to five minutes into your workout as you feel your heart rate start to rise and you start to breathe harder. Check at regular intervals.

BEGINNER CARDIO PROGRAMME
Note that the levels given refer to your cardiovascular practice not your Pilates level of ability. If you are new to aerobic-style workouts, please start slowly. Nothing will put you off more than an injury from doing too much too soon. To further prevent injury, remember that you will need to warm up and cool down before and after your cardio workout. If you are able to find somewhere to lie down, Spine Curls with Scarf (page 52) is great for this, otherwise try:

Walking on the Spot (page 135)
Standing Side Reach with Knee Bends (page 92)
Standing Quadriceps Stretch (page 134)
Shoulder Stretch (page 137)
As a cool down once your body is warm: Hip Flexor and Hamstring Stretch (page 88)

walking

Probably the best way to add more aerobic activity into your schedule is by doing brisk walking. Here's how to make it more of a structured part of your programme. Start gently with four walking sessions per week (note that only eight minutes of this initial session is aerobic).

1. Do five minutes of Pilates stretches to warm up (see above).
2. Walk slowly for a few minutes to get into your stride.
3. Walk briskly for 8 minutes.
4. Walk slowly for 5 minutes.
5. Stretch for 2 minutes to wind down.

Then each week, start to increase the amount of time that you are walking briskly until it reaches about 20 minutes. Top and tail as above with gentle stretches. Make sure that when you are brisk walking, your heart rate has been raised sufficiently. The intensity level should be 50–69 per cent of your maximum heart rate (see page 141). Carry on at this level for a few weeks until you feel that it has become much easier, that is, you do not feel tired after the workout or so breathless during the workout. Then you are ready to increase the pace and length of the workouts.

a beginner's sample week

In this sample week, I have added your Pilates practice. Notice that in the first session, I have used Pilates as the warm up and cool down. In this case, you could use any Pilates session from the workouts chapter (page 108).

Day One:	30 minutes Pilates. 20 minutes brisk walking. 15 minutes Pilates.
Day Two:	30 minutes home aerobic exercise DVD. 15 minutes Pilates.
Day Three:	20 minutes brisk walking. 30 minutes Pilates.
Day Four:	15 minutes Pilates. 20 minutes brisk walking.
Day Five:	30 minutes cumulative brisk walking.
Day Six:	20 minutes cycling or swimming. One hour Pilates session.
Day off	

INTERMEDIATE CARDIO PROGRAMME

As you become fitter, you should find that, as you exercise, your heart rate will decrease and your breathing will become easier. Eventually you will reach a point where your routine no longer raises your heart rate. This is when you should increase the intensity at which you are working. You can follow a similar outline as before or try 4 x 45-minute cardio workouts per week, exercising at moderate intensity, that is 50–70 per cent of your maximum heart rate. This time though, you should start to add some bouts of higher intensity work. For example, your brisk walking would be interspersed with some jogging.

1. Stretch for 5 minutes
2. Walk briskly for 5 minutes
3. Jog for 1 minute
4. Walk for 5 minutes

5. Jog for 1 minute
6. Walk slowly for 3 minutes
7. Stretch for 2 minutes

Then, as this becomes more comfortable, gradually increase the amount of time that you are jogging rather than walking briskly. Supplement the above with other cardio activities from the list as before.

ADVANCED CARDIO PROGRAMME

I would recommend increasing the intensity, rather than length or frequency, of your workouts. To do this, follow the guidelines before but include two interval training workouts. Interval training will increase the amount of calories you burn. It involves periods of high-intensity effort, followed by a recovery period of less intense physical activity. This stop-start approach has been shown to improve endurance and temporarily increase your metabolic rate after you stop exercising. For example, a 30-minute interval training session on a treadmill would look like the table below. Again, you may supplement your interval training for other cardio activities.

MINUTES	PACE	HEART RATE FOR ADVANCED
0–5	Warm up pace	60–70 per cent
5–7	Increase pace	70–80 per cent
7–11	Maintain steady pace	75–80 per cent
11–12	Brisk pace into high pace	85–95 per cent
12–14	Slower pace	75 per cent
14–15.30	High pace	85–95 per cent
15.30–17.30	Slower pace	75 per cent
17.30–19.15	High pace	85–95 per cent
19.15–21.15	Slower pace	75 per cent
21.15–25	High pace into brisk pace	75–95 per cent
25–30	Cool down pace	60–65 per cent

eating well

Remember that we are aiming not just for weight loss, but also for optimal health. A healthy, balanced diet can help to protect against heart disease and cancer. It can give your immune system a boost, helping to improve your resistance to colds and other infections. A healthy diet will ensure that you have the right energy levels to undertake the extra exercise that you have planned. It helps you to cope better with the stresses and strains of modern living.

As we saw in the opening chapters, losing weight depends on the very simple equation of burning more energy than you consume. While the weight-loss Pilates exercises and your cardiovascular activities will help to increase the 'energy out' part of the equation, we need now to ensure that the 'energy in' is sufficient to your needs.

Most diets boil down to the same thing – they get you to eat less. Whether they do this by cutting down on or cutting out carbohydrates, counting calories, eating solely fruit or vegetables or separating protein and carbohydrates, at the end of the day you will have less food on your plate. This means that you will lose weight. Initially at least.

But how often though do these diets prove to be disappointing? This is usually because that initial weight loss is due not to fat loss, but fluid loss. When you eat fewer calories, you cause the body to call on its reserves to release glycogen, which is then used for energy. Stored in the liver and lean muscle tissue, glycogen is held in a water base. The initial weight loss that you have early on in a diet is really just a loss of fluid. This is why the weight loss is temporary. If you continue to eat a severely restricted diet over a long period of time, your body starts to think that there might be a famine around the corner, so, to survive, it will start to 'hold onto' any food or drink you consume! Basically this is what happens when you find that the initial weight loss is followed by a 'plateau' when you struggle to lose more weight. I would like you to stop thinking of dieting and start thinking instead about good nutrition.

The extra exercise that you will be doing will probably mean that your appetite increases. Bearing in mind the energy in, energy out equation, you are going to need to keep an eye on the size of the portions you are eating. Opposite, I have given you approximate serving sizes but these are just to give you an idea of how much to eat. Once you have that image in mind, you should not feel the need to weigh every mouthful.

If you decide to count calories, then aim for approximately ten times your body weight in pounds for calories and divide this across your regular meals. Remember that 1lb (0.5kg) of body fat contains about 3,500 calories so, to lose 1lb in one week (which is healthy), you need to cut back 500 calories per day (7 x 500 = 3,500). Fortunately, many foods these days have the calories, fat content, etc on the labelling.

fruit and vegetables

Normal guidelines recommend five portions of fruit or vegetables a day. They are so good for you, providing vitamins and minerals, dietary fibre and phytochemicals that help to protect against certain diseases. The World Cancer Research Fund (WCRF) estimates that a diet rich in a variety of fruit and vegetables could prevent 20 per cent of all cancers. The nutrients help to support the thyroid gland and this will, in turn, help you to maintain a healthy metabolic rate. They also contain fibre which helps to remove excess fats from the body and are packed with anti-ageing antioxidants.

When choosing your fruit and vegetables, aim to eat as many different colours as possible – that way you can be assured of obtaining the widest range of nutrients. Think of all the colourful varieties: blueberries, strawberries, apricots, kiwi fruit, peaches, oranges, beetroot, broccoli and spinach. Do include at least two portions of dark green vegetables per day.

Try also to pick seasonal local produce. Having said that, frozen fruits and vegetables are a great standby and very convenient. Similarly, canned fruits and vegetables are useful to have in your store cupboard but be sure that they are canned in natural juices not sugary syrups and note any salt added. Dried fruits will count towards your daily quota. Juices are great. Smoothies are increasingly popular and taste fantastic but just be aware that they may be high in calories. Read the labels too on fruit drinks which are often loaded with sugar.

Raw is normally best, when appropriate and feasible. An unpeeled raw apple is going to have more nutrients than a peeled or cooked one. If you need to peel fruit and vegetables, try to peel as thinly as possible as a lot of the goodness is just below the skin and may be lost otherwise. Some fruits and vegetables, of course, must be cooked. Lightly steaming is best to retain as much of the natural goodness as possible, then poaching, baking or grilling.

What counts as one portion?

1 apple, peach, pear

2 plums, kiwis, or satsuma

1 cup (100g) berries or grapes

Small glass (150ml) of unsweetened fruit juice

2 tablespoon (90g) cooked vegetables

1 tablespoon dried fruits

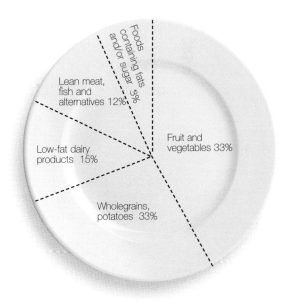

Foods containing fats and/or sugar 3%

Lean meat, fish and alternatives 12%

Fruit and vegetables 33%

Low-fat dairy products 15%

Wholegrains, potatoes 33%

wholegrains and starchy vegetables

This food group includes complex or starchy carbohydrates such as rice, bread, pasta, muesli and other breakfast cereals, potatoes and corn. The grains you use should be wholegrains, which are a source of complex carbohydrates and provide dietary fibre, protein, vitamins and minerals, but their main job is to provide energy. By choosing fibre-rich wholegrains rather than refined grains, you will receive slow-release energy which helps to keep blood sugar levels stable. High-fibre foods are filling which means they help you to feel full more quickly and prevent you from feeling hungry for longer.

Processing or refining food robs it of valuable nutrients. If you take wheat, for example, the process of refining wheat into white flour destroys over 19 nutrients as well as eliminating valuable dietary fibre. You will need to clear your cupboard of refined grains, cakes, biscuits and snack foods and stock up instead on wholegrains such as oats, brown rice, whole wheat, granary flours, whole spelt flour, 'wholemeal' couscous, millet and quinoa.

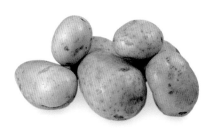

Depending on your appetite and calorie requirement, aim to eat about six servings from this group each day. One serving equals:
3 tablespoons wholegrain breakfast cereal (e.g. muesli, porridge)
1 slice wholegrain bread (granary is a great choice)
2 heaped tablespoons boiled brown rice (brown basmati tastes best)
3 heaped tablespoons pasta
2 medium-sized potatoes (preferably boiled new potatoes with their skins intact or a small baked potato in its jacket)

lean meat, fish and other proteins

Food from this group should form 12 per cent of your total food intake. This group provides protein, essential for the maintenance and repair of cells and for the production of enzymes, antibodies and hormones. Good sources include lean meat, fish, eggs, beans and pulses, nuts and seeds.

If you choose meat as your protein source, wherever possible, buy the best cuts available. Trim away visible fat before cooking. Chicken should ideally be free-range, as should eggs. It is advisable to take the skin off chicken portions to reduce the fat content.

Be sure to eat at least three portions of fish a week, two of which should be oily fish, such as salmon, sardines, mackerel and fresh tuna which are vital sources of the omega fatty acids, something that cannot be manufactured by the body. It is the long chain omega 3s, EPA and DHA that are the ones found mostly in oily fish. They have two distinct roles: to aid the growth, development and function of the brain and central nervous system and to help with the regulation of chemical processes which, in turn, helps to relieve the symptoms of a wide range of health problems and also to prevent them in the first place. They have anti-inflammatory properties, are good for joints and have been shown to help reduce the risk of heart disease and strokes by helping to reduce cholesterol levels in the blood and making the blood less sticky and less likely to clot.

Aim to eat between two and four servings from this group a day. One serving equals approximately:
90g lean red meat
125g chicken, skin removed
125g–150g fish
2 eggs
2 tablespoons nuts or seeds

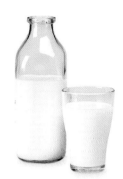

dairy products

Dairy products should make up 15 per cent of your daily diet. They are an important source of calcium, essential for strong bones and teeth.

Unfortunately, many foods in this group tend to be high in saturated fat. For years, a diet high in saturated fat, like butter, has been associated with high levels of potentially harmful LDL cholesterol in the blood. This, in turn, has been seen as a trigger for heart disease. If you wish to lose weight and keep your heart healthy, you will certainly need to avoid eating a lot of saturated fat.

However, studies have questioned the assumption that substituting butter for margarine is a healthier option. Recent reports have revealed that the real villain of the piece are trans fats. Trans fats not only raise bad cholesterol levels, they also lower good cholesterol! Trans fats are formed when oil is hydrogenated or processed to become solid. As they are cheap to produce and help to prolong shelf life, they are found in many processed foods, especially margarine, fried foods, biscuits, cakes, take-aways, ready-meals and many other baked goods. Try to avoid these.

Aim to eat between two and three portions from this group a day. One portion equals:
1 glass of semi-skimmed milk
150g carton of yoghurt
100g cottage cheese or 40g hard full-fat cheese such as Cheddar

the importance of essential fats and oils

We have seen that not all fat is bad. We need essential fatty acids (EFAs) to help us to manage our weight and maintain our health. They are particularly important for the health of the skin. As well as oily fish, essential fats can also be found in nuts and seeds, vegetables, grains, beans, and certain oils such as rapeseed, walnut and flax-seed oil.

EFAs are important for transporting stored fats out of the adipose tissues. All cells in the body have a fatty layer that protects them from potential damage, allowing nutrients in and waste matter out! This fatty layer is made up of essential fatty acids. If your diet is deficient in these fats, the cell walls become too rigid, preventing toxins, such as stored fats, from escaping. The fat becomes denser and harder to budge. Limit your total fat consumption to under 20 grams per day. Go for the good essential fatty acids found in fish, seeds, nuts and beans.

watch your sugar intake

As sugar provides very little real nutritional value and empty calories, it makes sense to cut down on it wherever you can. What we really need to do is re-educate our palate. If you need to sweeten food, try adding fruit or a little honey. A grated pear or a handful of berries, for example, will naturally sweeten a bowl of porridge or yoghurt while also adding valuable nutrients.

watch your salt intake

Although salt, whose technical name is sodium chloride, plays a vital role in the body's fluid balance, muscle and nerve activity, almost all of us consume far more of it than we actually need or is good for us. Experts recommend that we limit our intake of salt to no more than 6g a day (equivalent to about 2.4g sodium). Eating too much salt has been implicated as the cause of many health problems, including high blood pressure, which in turn increases the risk of stroke and heart disease. It may cause leeching of calcium from the bones, increasing the risk of osteoporosis. It has also been linked to an increased risk of stomach cancer. Around 80 per cent of the sodium in our diet comes from processed foods, so it is important to read food labels properly and steer clear of those with a high salt content.

the glycaemic index and glycaemic load

The Glycaemic Index (GI) ranks foods according to how quickly they can be digested and converted into glucose. Foods with a high GI rating cause a rapid rise in blood sugar levels, those with a low GI rating result in a steadier, gradual rise. A diet rich in refined products such as white flour, sugar, biscuits and so on would result in quick surges of energy that soon subside leaving the body craving its next fix! Research shows that low GI diets help to control diabetes by improving blood sugar levels and fat metabolism. They may also help to prevent the onset of Type 2 diabetes. While it used to be thought that people with diabetes were the only ones who had to think about blood sugar levels, there is growing evidence that everyone should be concerned about keeping blood sugars under control to help prevent chronic disease and manage weight.

By including low GI foods in your diet, foods such as oats, pulses and vegetables, you can provide a more constant supply of energy. Fortunately, most healthy foods have a low GI rating. There are, however, some exceptions: bananas, carrots and potatoes for example. The problem with the GI index is that it compares an amount of food containing a set amount of carbohydrate (50g) against a standard, without regard for the typical portion size. Carrots, as I mentioned, have a high GI rating but you would have to eat seven to get 50g worth of carbohydrate. There is a new measure called the Glycaemic Load (GL) which is based on the GI but takes into account portion sizes when ranking food. On the GL table carrots fare better. Eating foods with a low GL will help prevent energy dips.

eat at regular intervals

Try not to leave more than three to four hours between meals and never skip meals. Breakfast is particularly important. If you allow yourself to get too hungry, you are more likely to over-eat later. Some people thrive best on getting the majority of their daily calories in three square meals, others do better with the 'grazing' approach, eating little and often. Try both and see what suits you.

know your portion size

Keep in mind the portion sizes listed previously. Take your time eating and stop before you feel full or bloated. It takes time for your body to register that you have eaten enough. Also make sure that you chew your food thoroughly. If you do not chew your food properly before you swallow, it will mean that there is a reduced surface area that is exposed for your digestive enzymes to act, making digestion harder

keep a record

Actually writing down what you eat on a daily basis is a great way to ensure you stick to your healthy-eating regime. It will help to highlight any particular weaknesses you may have in your diet and areas you may need to improve.

limit your intake of alcohol

Studies have shown that red wine, in particular, has numerous health benefits as it contains natural plant chemicals, polyphenols, which can protect against the danger of heart disease, strokes, diabetes and certain cancers. But how much alcohol should we be drinking?

In the UK it is advised that men should not regularly drink more than three to four units a day and women should not drink more than two to three. The key, however, is to know what constitutes a unit and to understand that the number of recommended units can change over time to reflect trends in drinking patterns – for example, more red wine of a higher alcohol content (such as Shiraz) is being drunk in the UK than ever before.

Two to three units can be consumed in just one standard glass (175ml) of Shiraz Cabernet red wine (typically 2.3 units) or of Chardonnay or Pinot Grigio (typically 2.1 units). A large 250ml glass offered by many restaurants would constitute 3.1 units for a typical Merlot and 3.3 units for Shiraz Cabernet! Two single gin and tonics would typically total 2.6 units.

The key is to stay fully aware of the amount of alcohol that you consume and to recognise just how easy it is for those units to creep up. When thinking about weight loss, we need to remember that alcohol contains a significant number of calories. It can also stimulate the biochemical pathways involved in appetite control, which means that after too much alcohol you can easily end up over-eating. And, finally, alcohol can slow down fat metabolism and make it harder to lose weight. Having a few alcohol-free days each week will help to keep your intake down.

eating out

If you only eat out occasionally, then, in my opinion, you should relax and enjoy yourself and choose what you want from the menu. You can always burn a few extra calories the next day by briskly walking a few more miles! But if you eat out on a regular basis, you need to learn how to navigate your way around a menu so that you stay within your healthy-eating guidelines.

Because you are probably going to be eating more than normal during the meal, you'd do best to avoid the bread basket. Most restaurants have salads now as a first course and if you ask for the salad dressing on the side, you can add just a little for flavour. The main course is easy, lean, grilled meat or fish with vegetables. Vegetarian options are often limited but as long as you avoid creamy or heavy cheese sauces you should be fine. Again, ask for rice or boiled potatoes on the side so that you can control your portion size. For dessert, unless there is fruit on the menu, I'd go straight to coffee or tea. Watch the alcohol intake when you are out, it's easy for it to creep up and then have all your good intentions disappear!

avoid getting constipated

We need fibre to keep our digestive tract healthy. There are two types of fibre – insoluble fibre and soluble fibre. We need both. Insoluble fibre is found mainly in wholegrain cereals, fruit and vegetables and pulses. It has the effect of holding or absorbing water, making stools larger, softer and easier to pass. Insoluble fibre also speeds up the rate at which waste material is passed thorough the body. This process is believed to play an important role in preventing bowel cancer by reducing the length of time cancer-causing toxins stay within the system. Soluble fibre, found in oats and oat bran, beans and pulses and some fruits can help to lower high blood cholesterol levels and slow the absorption of sugar into the blood stream. The recommended intake of fibre for men and women is 18g a day.

drink enough water to stay hydrated

Water is vital for transporting and burning fat. As you exercise more, it becomes even more important for eliminating those waste products that result from your improved metabolic activity. Most experts recommend drinking between eight to ten glasses a day. You can obtain a lot of hydration from fruit and vegetables but you will probably still need to actually drink eight to ten glasses. Thirst, sadly, is not a reliable indicator of how much water you need. One way to check that you are drinking enough is to keep an eye on your urine. It should be pale in colour rather than dark.

lifestyle choices

In this section, we will be examining some alternative approaches to losing weight and also some surprising new research into why some people have found that, in spite of following all the rules, the weight simply will not shift. In some cases, there might be one factor of your lifestyle that is preventing you from making progress.

are you getting enough sleep'?

Doctors have known for some time now that many hormones are affected by sleep. Recently research has highlighted the hormones leptin and ghrelin as influencing our appetite. Studies have shown that the production of both may be influenced by how much or how little we sleep.

These two hormones work together to control our feelings of hunger and satiety. Ghrelin, which is produced in the gastrointestinal tract, stimulates our appetite. Leptin, produced in our fat cells, sends signals to our brain to indicate when we are full up. If you fail to get enough sleep, your leptin levels can drop, this means that you may still feel hungry despite the fact that you have eaten sufficient quantities of food. At the same time, lack of sleep causes ghrelin levels in the body to rise, thus stimulating your appetite, leaving you wanting more food.

The quality of sleep counts too. Studies have shown that a decreased amount of time spent in restorative deep or slow-wave sleep has been associated with significantly-reduced levels of growth hormone. Growth hormone is a protein that helps the body to regulate the proportions of fat and muscle in adults. How much sleep do you need? Well, researchers agree that the optimum amount of sleep for each person varies. Some people can thrive on six hours a night, while others need eight or even nine hours. Only you can tell whether you are getting enough. Joseph Pilates extolled the virtues of a good night's sleep. He felt that amongst the most important requirements for a good night's sleep are quiet, darkness, fresh air and mental calm.

do you have too much stress in your life?

Even if you are getting enough sleep at night, it is still possible that chronic stress is affecting your health and your weight. Stress itself is not bad. It is a basic survival tool, a response to potential danger. The problem with modern society is that the type of stress that we meet has changed. While we might still be occasionally subjected to a life-threatening event, where the fight or flight response would save our lives, many of us are also under chronic stress. This may be from working long hours, financial problems, marital problems, or worrying about the kids.

This kind of chronic stress weakens your immune system, accelerates ageing and, importantly for us here, can cause metabolic changes that lead to weight gain. Perhaps you are the kind of person who is 'on the go' all day every day. You would think that being busy all the time would help weight loss but instead chronic stress interferes with your hunger and satiety messengers, making you crave certain foods. And, sadly, it is not broccoli we crave when we are stressed!

Stress encourages our body to store the extra calories as fat. The body 'believes' that the fact that you are stressed indicates hard times ahead, perhaps famine? Better store some fat just in case. If this state of chronic stress continues, you leave yourself open to increased risk of obesity, Type 2 diabetes, high blood pressure and heart disease.

try the following stress busters:

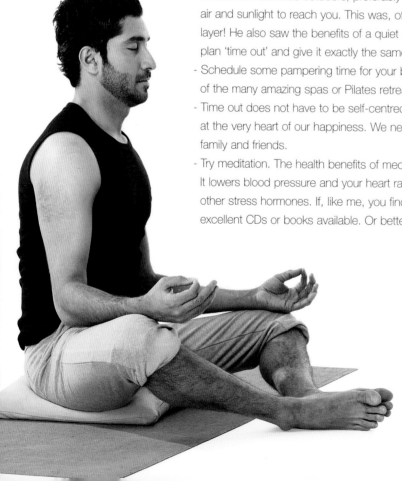

- Joseph Pilates wrote of the importance of balancing the intense concentration of our work by embracing every form of 'pleasurable living'. He was passionate about taking recreational activities outdoors, preferably wearing as little as possible to allow the fresh air and sunlight to reach you. This was, of course, when there was more of an ozone layer! He also saw the benefits of a quiet night in. What matters, I believe, is that we plan 'time out' and give it exactly the same priority as an important meeting in the diary.
- Schedule some pampering time for your body. If you can afford it, plan a break at one of the many amazing spas or Pilates retreats cropping up around the world.
- Time out does not have to be self-centred. Our relationships with the people we love lie at the very heart of our happiness. We need to put time and effort into connecting with family and friends.
- Try meditation. The health benefits of meditation are almost too numerous to mention. It lowers blood pressure and your heart rate, and reduces the amount of cortisol and other stress hormones. If, like me, you find meditation challenging, try one of the excellent CDs or books available. Or better still, find a teacher!

Aim to meditate for 15 to 20 minutes a day. Try this simple meditation:

- Find a quiet place where you will not be disturbed. The room should be warm, softly lit and well-ventilated.
- Sit comfortably on a chair, with both feet on the floor or sit cross legged if you are comfortable.
- Close your eyes and relax your jaw and face muscles. Allow your tongue to widen at its base.
- Bring your awareness to your breath, to its gentle ebb and flow. Feel your abdomen expand as you inhale.
- Gently allow the breath to flow out through the mouth. Make your exhalation twice as long as your inhalation. Empty your lungs. Feel the new breath fill your lungs. Breathe slowly. Count as you inhale and exhale.
- One by one, empty your mind of the worries accumulated during the day until you can focus on a single positive thought, image or affirmation.
- If you like, you may repeat the ancient Sanskrit mantra 'om' (a long drawn-out sound that reverberates through you).
- When you are ready, gradually become aware of your surroundings...first the sounds, the smells and then the sights around you. Move your body and stand slowly.

regular health checks

The importance of regular health checks appropriate to your age cannot be over emphasised. Joseph Pilates considered them a vital part of a healthy lifestyle and recommended regular physical check-ups every three months if you are over the age of 40. I'm not sure that our National Health Service will stretch to this but you should consult your doctor before you start exercising and this might be the perfect time to find out if you are due to have any particular check-ups. Dental health also has a direct bearing on your overall health, so don't forget to also see your dentist for regular check-ups.

increasing the variety and intensity of your pilates workouts

In this section, I want to look at ways in which you can maximise your weight loss by adding extra challenge to your Pilates practice. These 'tricks of the trade' not only make you work a little harder, they also help you to develop your mind-body connection, they add variety and, in the case of the stability apparatus, they add an extra element of fun to your workouts!

You should be familiar with all the exercises in the Fundamentals and All Levels sections before you attempt any of the following.

change the breathing pattern

Co-ordinating the breath with the movement is probably one of the most difficult skills you have to learn with your Pilates practice. Once you have it mastered, there is a great deal of satisfaction to be had from the perfect execution of an exercise. It is at this point, when you are safe within your 'comfort zone', that it can be a good idea to, on occasion, change the breathing pattern.

It is not appropriate with every exercise, but you could try adding an extra breath when you are in the final part of the movement just before the return. This will mean that your muscles will need to 'hold' you in this position for a second or two longer, thus working them a fraction harder. But note that Pilates is in its essence about movement, not 'holding positions', so only try this occasionally and only add one extra breath…no more.

change the pace

By now it should be no surprise that I am not going to tell you to speed it up – I am going to tell you to slow it down. By doing an exercise at a slower pace your muscles really have to work hard to keep control of the movement. When you try this, you will have to add an extra breath as you make the movements. Note that this is different to the advice given above where you added an extra breath at the top of the movement. In this case, you will still be moving as you add an extra breath.

focus on the return phase of the exercise

If you are practising your Pilates correctly, you will always stay mindful of all your movements from the first breath in the starting position, right through to the last breath as you return to the mat. The return phase of each exercise is very important. You would never simply collapse back onto the mat – the return needs to be controlled. You might like, however, to give the return phase extra consideration. It may not increase the intensity of what you are doing but it will help to improve your technique and ensure that you get every last 'ounce' of benefit from the exercise.

investing in home studio accessories

I have always been passionate about Pilates matwork. I love the studio equipment, but the fact that the mat exercises can be done anywhere without any expensive equipment has inspired me to spread the word. Having said this, I am now going to tell you about some home equipment you can buy! You do not need any of these, but they are fun. See page 158 for stockists.

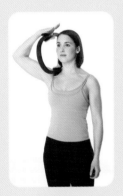

toning circle

Created by Joseph Pilates and also known as 'Magic Circles', these can be used to add extra strength work and resistance to Pilates exercises when working with the arms or legs. They are unbelievably effective at toning the inner thighs and upper arms – if these are your problem areas, they are certainly worth the investment. See the photos on the left for examples of how to use a toning circle.

stability products

We are spoilt now by the wide range of stability products that are available, all of which are great fun to work with. Their 'instability' makes you work your deep core muscles naturally. Please use these valuable tools with caution. I wholeheartedly recommend that you find a qualified Body Control Pilates teacher to help to show you how to gain maximum benefit and to use them safely. In the meantime, here are a few ideas to inspire you to find out more.

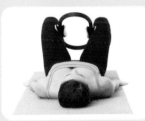

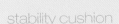

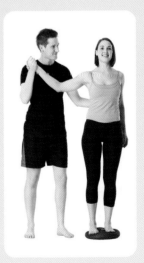

stability cushion

These take many forms – the most popular is called a 'Sitfit'. With a diameter of typically about 33cm, they are essentially an inflated circular cushion made from rubber. Great for sitting on to improve posture and strengthen the back and abdominal muscles, they are also fun to stand on to challenge and improve balance and proprioception!

wobble board

Exercising with a wooden wobble board is generally regarded by our teachers and clients as the best way to prepare for the ski slopes. A wobble board is essentially a standing platform sitting on two rockers. They help you to work on your balance, alignment, ankle mobility, Achilles tendon length, arches of the foot and your overall posture and balance. I would suggest using a rectangular or square wobble board rather than a circular board, as they are more stable. For reasons of safety, look for a board with a non-slip surface and, when using the board, stand facing a wall or rail at arm's length so that you can support yourself if necessary.

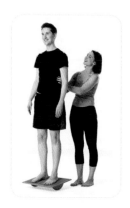

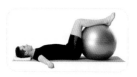

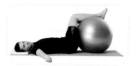

physioball

Also known as gym balls or Swiss balls, most fitness clubs and gyms have them, and certainly all Pilates studios use them regularly. They are also perfect to use at your desk instead of a chair, although for health and safety reasons, you should sit them in a base to secure them. Please make sure you buy the right one for your height.

height	ball size
Under 5ft	45cm
5'0"–5'8"	55cm
5'9"–6'3"	65cm
Over 6'3"	75cm

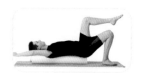

foam roller

Another popular addition to Pilates classes has been the foam roller. Unlike the balls, the roller supports the whole length of your spine and is great for challenging your stability. You can buy half rollers and large and small diameter rollers. If you are fit, with no medical problems, I would recommend starting with the larger roller.

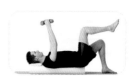

triad ball™

These are my personal favourite as they mould their shape to the curves in your spine perfectly and are a great way of building more core strength and flexibility. Blow the ball up so that it is not quite fully inflated – it will take you less than 30 seconds! They are also incredibly portable as they deflate easily. I keep one in my suitcase for use whenever I'm travelling.

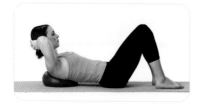

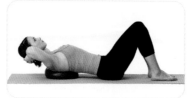

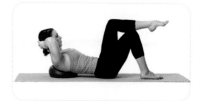

maintaining your weight

What next? I am hoping that, although you have now reached your ideal weight, you will not want to give up your Pilates practice, cardio activities or stop eating well. You should be feeling great as well as looking great. Our goal was never just weight loss but optimal health. Cast your mind back to how you felt before you started this programme and notice the difference.

This weight-loss programme has given you many skills to enable you to live a healthy life. Continue to follow the guidelines, but now that weight loss is no longer your goal, you can relax a little. Do not worry if, occasionally, you miss a Pilates session you had planned or fail to reach your 10,000 steps a day. Try to do a minimum of two hours Pilates per week.

You will still have to maintain your heart health by doing aerobic activities for a minimum of 30 minutes on five days each week or more vigorous intensity aerobic physical activity for a minimum of 20 minutes on three days a week. By now, I suspect that these will have become part of your lifestyle and you will be thoroughly enjoying them. Remember, though, if you over-train, you will stress your body and it will not have time to heal itself.

If you feel that you need to progress more, consider purchasing some of the items on pages 155–156. You might also try enrolling in classes with a qualified teacher or even trying a Pilates studio where you can work out on some of the amazing equipment that Joseph Pilates designed.

With regards to your diet, some people can maintain their weight even if they eat more; others will need to watch what they eat more closely. Keep an eye on your weight, your BMI and your waist-to-hip ratio and stay within healthy guidelines. Be sure that you do not drop below or go above these. The energy equation still applies. If you eat more calories than you burn, your weight will start to creep up again. Healthy eating will probably have changed your tastebuds. I find now that I simply do not want to eat junk food at all; the desire has completely gone. But just as you can occasionally skip a Pilates session, so too the occasional 'slip' will do you no harm.

And finally, if you have followed the weight-loss programme and achieved your target weight, or even if you have made some progress towards your goals, congratulations! Take a moment and consider just how much you have learned about your body and how much you have achieved. You did this, no one else. This book merely gave you the tools you needed but you took responsibility for your own health and fitness. Well done!

further information

Pilates information, teachers and equipment

Body Control Pilates
Association
www.bodycontrol.co.uk
www.bodycontrolpilates.com

UK Register of Exercise
Professionals
www.exerciseregister.org

Pilates Home Accessories
www.bodycontrol.co.uk

Foam Rollers (Fit Roll)
www.sisseluk.com

MBT Physiological footwear
www.swissmasai.co.uk

Swopper seats
www.swopper-uk.com

Pedometers
www.amazon.co.uk

Nutrition

UK Food Standards Agency
www.eatwell.gov.uk/healthydiet

British Nutrition Foundation
www.nutrition.org.uk

beat (Beating Eating
Disorders)
www.b-eat.co.uk

NHS Direct
www.nhsdirect.nhs.uk

National Obesity Forum
www.nationalobesityforum.org.uk

Department of Health
www.dh.gov.uk

Other

Charted Society of
Physiotherapists
www.csp.org.uk

Chartered Physiotherapists in
Women's Health
www.acpwh.org.uk

General Chiropractic Council
www.gcc-uk.org

General Osteopathic Council
www.osteopathy.org.uk

British Meditation Society
www.britishmeditationsociety.org

index